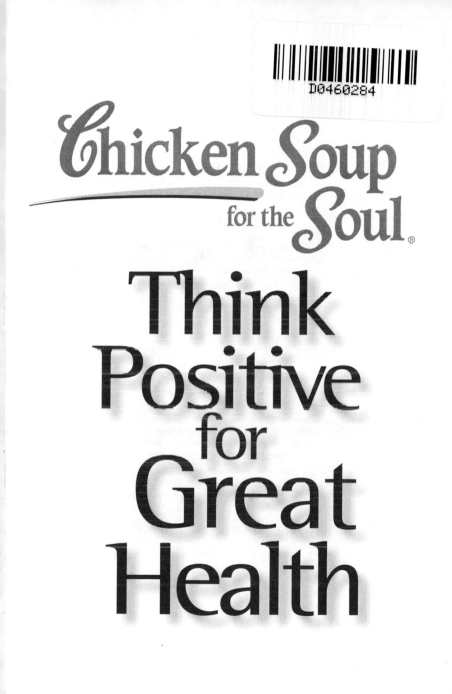

Chicken Soup for the Soul.

Think Positive for Great Health

Chicken Soup for the Soul: Think Positive for Great Health
Use Your Mind to Promote Your Own Healing and Wellness
Dr. Jeff Brown

Published by Chicken Soup for the Soul Health, an imprint of Chicken Soup for the Soul Publishing, LLC www.chickensoup.com

The publisher gratefully acknowledges the many publishers and individuals who granted Chicken Soup for the Soul permission to reprint the cited material.

This publication contains the opinions and ideas of the authors. It is intended to provide helpful and informative material on the subjects addressed in the publication. Harvard Medical School and the publisher are not engaged in rendering medical, health, psychological, or any other kind of personal professional services in the book. The reader should consult a health professional before adopting suggestions in this book.

Harvard Medical School, the authors and the publisher specifically disclaim all responsibility for any liability, loss, or risk, personal or otherwise, incurred as a direct or indirect consequence of the use and application of any of the contents of this book.

Front cover and interior photo courtesy of iStockphoto.com/Yuri_Arcurs (© Jacob Wackerhausen). Back cover photo of Dr. Jeff Brown © Eric Laurits.

Cover and Interior Design & Layout by Pneuma Books, LLC
For more info on Pneuma Books, visit www.pneumabooks.com

Distributed to the booktrade by Simon & Schuster. SAN: 200-2442

Publisher's Cataloging-In-Publication Data
(Prepared by The Donohue Group, Inc.)

Brown, Jeff, 1969-
   Chicken soup for the soul : think positive for great health : use your mind to promote your own healing and wellness / Jeff Brown.

   p. ; cm.

   Summary: A collection of stories accompanied by medical advice on the topics of using your mind to promote better health, how to find the right doctor, how to manage your medical situation, how to reduce stress and other factors that have a negative impact on health.
   ISBN: 978-1-935096-90-0

   1. Mind and body--Popular works. 2. Health--Popular works. 3. Stress management--Popular works. 4. Mind and body--Anecdotes. 5. Health--Anecdotes. 6. Stress management--Anecdotes. I. Title. II. Title: Think positive for great health

PN6071.M53 B76 2012

810.2/02/356/1   2012939987

PRINTED IN THE UNITED STATES OF AMERICA
on acid∞free paper

21 20 19 18 17 16 15 14 13 12   01 02 03 04 05 06 07 08 09 10

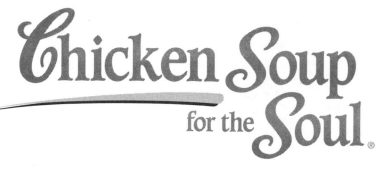

Chicken Soup for the Soul ®

Think Positive
for
Great Health

Use Your Mind to Promote Your Own Healing and Wellness

by DR. JEFF BROWN of HARVARD MEDICAL SCHOOL

Chicken Soup for the Soul Publishing, LLC
Cos Cob, CT

Chicken Soup

www.chickensoup.com

for the Soul

Contents

Chapter 3

～ Hope for the Best and *Expect* the Best ～

Chapter 4

Dr. Seuss, Kevorkian or Oz:
～ Connecting with the Right Doctor ～

Chapter 5
～ **Brain Strategies for Robust Living** ～

Chapter 6
～ **Increase Your Health IQ—Now!** ～

Chapter 7
⁓ Avoid the F-word: Frustration ⁓

Chapter 8
⁓ Tame the Anxiety Beast ⁓

Introduction

No one can afford to be sick, especially in the face of a lethargic economy and disgraceful healthcare costs. Conversation starters used to be about the weather, politics or religion. Now, outrageous healthcare costs are on the short list of what you'll find in common with people you hardly know.

According to a Kaiser Family Foundation statistic, employers were paying an average family insurance premium of $15,073 in 2011. Heated battles between patients and their insurance companies over ruthless denials of coverage, disgruntled providers who are being stripped financially by collapsing reimbursement rates, and those individuals who simply don't seek treatment because of high deductibles make for a perfect storm that's not going to be over soon. Have you noticed how your health has taken on a financial tone? General quality of life, contentment, and happiness should always be front and center, but advocating for your health has now become a financial preoccupation for many people. Let me be clear. Good health is now a commodity and is something you have to haggle over, rather than enjoy.

This unhealthy problem facing everyone won't fade. If your strategy has been to "wait it out," then wait no longer and start taking charge of your health. The responsibility of great health is falling to individuals more than ever in history. Not just caring about your health, but being in the driver's seat of your health, is one of newest, most vital responsibilities you face today and in the future.

A key ingredient in facing this responsibility of managing your health is your brain. This is where the good news comes in! Advancing research continues to expand knowledge and furthers understanding of the brain and its capacity to change and influence our thoughts, feelings, and behaviors. You are positioned better than ever to utilize your brain to improve your life. By the way, you already own your brain. It won't cost you a thing.

You can tap into your brain to maintain or improve your healthcare. Yes, it takes some good old-fashioned work ethic to apply principles and strategies, but your health is worth the effort. If change is on your horizon, you'll have to be the one to put it there. So, don't wait any longer to start changing. Use your brain to develop optimism and positive emotions. Use your brain to visualize recovery or conquering new health challenges. Use your brain to develop healthy mindsets and reduce frustration and anxiety. Build your knowledge of psychological principles that will allow you to make better decisions and develop new habits that can give you a healthy overhaul.

Chicken Soup for the Soul: Think Positive for Great Health has been written specifically with your brain and you in mind. Even a little interest in living a healthy life speaks volumes about your motives, hopes, and self-respect. You and your health can be companions for life.

~ Jeff Brown, Psy.D., ABPP, Psychologist ~

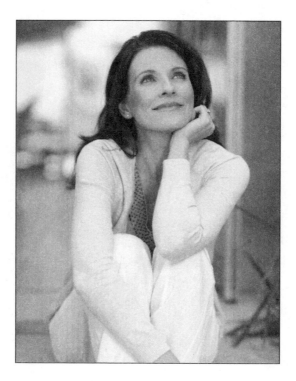

Chapter 1
Your Mind and Your Body: Best Friends for Life

Give Me a Break

In the summer after our tenth grade year, Sue, Louise and I were the three musketeers, the triangle offense, and Neapolitan ice cream. Neapolitan ice cream, not because we were Italian, but because Sue was a brunette, Louise a platinum blonde and I a redhead. All three of us sported long hair, great looking bodies in our hip huggers and crop tops, and as we strolled along the streets we counted the number of horn honks we received like notches on our belts. It was hot that summer and so were we.

That was the last summer we hung out like that, for in our eleventh grade year we could drive. And drive we did. We cruised the boulevard, pushed the pedal to the metal, triple-dated with boyfriends, raced to the beach, and brought all our friends, in the trunks of our parents' cars, to the drive-in movies. That was also the summer Sue began working and saving for college.

Sue lived with her aunt and uncle along with their two children. She knew no one would pay her way through college, unlike Louise and me, who already knew that our college tuitions were covered.

Sue scrimped and saved her money the summer before our senior year. She slaved away at several jobs from the end of school in June to the first day of school in September. Louise and I attended summer school and weren't as happy-go-lucky as our first summer together. Grades and SATs were important now. Louise and I ended up settling for a state college but Sue enrolled at the University of California at Los Angeles.

After high school graduation our lives rapidly changed. Louise and I learned that summer school was a nifty way of lightening our course load during the year as well as keeping up with our school credits. Sue still worked and economized from June until September. She lived in the dorms at UCLA. Even though she was only a fifteen-minute drive over the hill, we didn't see much of her. Occasionally we met in Westwood, near the university. It had to be close to Sue's dorm for she either worked, attended class or studied. Sue's college pattern: work-class-study.

Beginning our second year in college, I noticed another pattern in Sue's life. Since she had started working during the summers, back before our eleventh grade year, Sue had never taken a vacation. There were of course the weekends, but when college started, Sue labored those days as well. This was something we all knew, but didn't think about much. It just stuck in the back of our minds. When Louise and I considered a fun excursion, we knew Sue was toiling away at work.

The first time it happened, no one paid attention. Getting mononucleosis before school started our senior year in high school was no big deal. Everybody got mono back then—the kissing disease. Sue sweated and slept in bed for a week at the end of the summer, as school began. Louise and I teased her by telling our friends she needed to recover from being over-kissed. The next year, before college began, she contracted some kind of virus or flu again and had another sleep-filled, sweaty week in bed. She couldn't go to Yosemite with us. When it happened the third time, the same way the next year, it made sense to me. Sue had not taken a vacation, so her body did it for her. Fun holiday? No, but it was a break. She subconsciously managed the perfect body breakdown, missing only one week of work, each year, preceding school registration.

I visited Sue that September before our second year in college. "How are you feeling?" I asked, as I put flowers in a vase by her bed.

"We must really stop meeting like this," she moaned.

"Do you remember the first time you got sick?"

She thought for a second. "Yeah!" Her voice went up two octaves. "I felt embarrassed my first day back our senior year. You and Louise spread rumors about me being absent from school because I kissed dead people... or something like that."

"We were just being silly." I laughed. "I've been thinking about this. What has not happened in your life since that first summer of mono?" Putting her hand on her chin she thought. "Isn't it interesting you get sick every year right before school starts?" Her eyes opened wide as this new notion made sense to her. "Your body forced you on a vacation... in bed, every year before school started."

Her face lit up as she asked, "Wow! What do I do about it?"

"You take charge and decide when and where your next holiday is. Go on an exciting vacation!" I encouraged.

"Exciting and inexpensive," Sue retorted.

"Okay, do anything, go anywhere, see anyone, just take a

break!" I left her full of hope as she recuperated from her dis-ease. Dis-ease because her body was not in its normal state of peace and health. Her mind, preoccupied with worry about her finances, caused this illness in her body.

Next June, the summer of our third year in college, we talked about her mind-body connection again. During the year, Sue paid more attention to her body. She noticed that thoughts about money made her body feel rigid and hot, the way she felt before getting sick. In the past, she never realized a connection between what her mind thought and what her body felt. This year was different. She decided to break her pattern and join her family for a week in August at the beach. We both felt excited about the possibilities. The summer came and went without a sign of illness.

In September, Sue telephoned. "Debi, I never realized the power my mind had over my body. It knew I needed a break all those years. But I obsessed over money and grades, leaving no room for balance in my life."

A huge grin spread across my face as she shared her new insight. Sue yanked back control and smashed her cycle of work-class-study-flu, by taking a vacation! Her break from work and school helped Sue heal. She learned the importance her thoughts, either conscious or unconscious, and her self-talk had on the wellness of her body.

~ Deborah Ellis ~

Restoring
Body and Soul

My divorce thirty years ago left me more than heartsick, it left me sick in spirit. The first years as a single parent were lonely and frightening, my self-esteem falling to an all-time low. It wasn't long before I noticed a sharp rise in my blood pressure and more frequent headaches. The constant stress settled into my body, especially in my neck and across my shoulders and upper back. I felt like I was carrying the weight of the world on my shoulders. As my body aches increased, so did my feelings of despair and failure. When I signed up for life insurance and had a medical checkup my blood pressure was so dangerously high I was almost turned down. I was overwhelmed and my life reflected it.

One day I was visiting my parents and my dad told me how hard it was to see me so sad. "Your marriage was so unhappy, I was hoping that you would bounce back after your divorce. I think you've forgotten how to be happy. You have two terrific kids and a family that loves you. Why are you still so sad all the time?" my dad asked. I was surprised by the question, but more shocked because I had no answer. The question continued to haunt me as I drove home and later, after I put the children to bed, I made a cup of tea and began thinking about how to change my mental outlook.

There were certainly difficulties to overcome, but many things in my life were wonderful and I wasn't making time to enjoy them. I began to take walks with my sister, taking time to notice the simple beauty of a field of buttercups or the sight of Mount Rainier on a clear summer day. Beauty was all around me, but I was so self-absorbed I no longer noticed. I began to spend more time laughing with my children and seeking activities we could enjoy together within our limited budget. My headaches became less frequent and my blood pressure slowly improved.

At a meeting with the pastor of my church, I told him how I had gotten into such a terrible depression and mentioned to him that I felt it would be good for me to do some kind of volunteer work. "I think it will help me to get outside of myself and look at the bigger picture," I told him. He thought it was a good idea and encouraged me to do some volunteer work with the church's youth. It was fun to work with the teenagers, helping them to put on plays for special events. Their sense of humor and high spirits lifted my mood.

As my outlook became more positive I became more interested in exercise and healthy eating. I took a beginning yoga class, trying to get back the flexibility I had when I was younger. I had always wanted to learn to tap dance, so at the age of forty I signed up for a beginning tap class for adults. Each new adventure brought more people into my life and I found new confidence. It wasn't an immediate transformation for me, but a steady improvement. For the first time in years I was having fun.

My health continued to improve, my blood pressure returned to normal, and my headaches became infrequent and less intense. I began hiking and camping with my children, an activity we had enjoyed before the divorce, which took us out into the fresh air and helped us bond as a family. The hiking increased my stamina, leaving me feeling strong and empowered. My tense body eased and I began to feel like the person I once was, only new and improved.

My health has continued to be strong, although a traumatic car accident did set me back a bit several years ago. I battled through that difficult time, learning anew the power of accepting what I cannot change and appreciating the good things that make up the majority of my life. One of the nicest things about changing my life was the number of people who were inspired to do the same thing. It is my experience that when you begin to live in a more positive frame of mind, that positive outlook spreads to others. Not only has my health benefited from thinking positively, my life growing richer and more fulfilling, but others around me have found greater joy as well. Believing in the power of positive can heal your body and restore your spirit.

~ Beth Arvin ~

Serving
Two Masters

For years I dreamed of becoming a healthcare executive. I finally got my coveted promotion to Vice President at age thirty-nine. My previous education and training were focused on this goal. The greater challenge came when, having married for the first time in my late thirties, I had our only child just a month shy of my forty-second birthday. Thus began my late-in-life, corporate mom boomerang from happy and prosperous to unhappy and unhealthy... and back to hope and healing.

Life stirred in our newly built suburban home by dawn each day. Meredith still needed help with dressing and meals. A last minute check of her book bag confirmed all forms were signed and lunch was safely tucked inside. Breakfast might be served in my stockings before I grabbed my heels and blazer.

On good days we had time to walk to school, Meredith's preference, while late starts required a drive. Her father or grandmother met her after classes and oversaw evening activities such as bathing and homework. Corporate expectations meant late nights and out-of-town travel for me. I had worked hard to attain my professional status and enjoyed the thrill of success, but it came with board meetings and business deals, which came with high priced, high calorie business dinners.

Being a full-time mom and full-time executive stressed my body, mind, and spirit more than I realized. Within a few years I found myself bloated, perpetually tired, and frequently depressed. The migraine headaches from two decades before returned. The familiar rash around my neck defied cortisone, leaving me splotchy and itchy. The joy of conquering new business horizons started to seem lower priority when Meredith was waiting up at night just to see her mom. Someone else fed her, gave her a bath, and read her nighttime stories, not me. Most days my mind and body ached from mixed loyalties.

Though I spoke at local seminars on how to be a super-woman/supermom, inside I knew my health and state of mind were far from super. I needed to decide what I really wanted in my life and go for it. "No one can serve two masters" was what the scripture told me (Matthew 6:24). Although I did not want to believe this, my body and spirit knew it. Something had to change. What bought me the most joy and peace was not my job.

"I know we need the money, but Meredith also needs a mom—a healthy one who can help her grow up," I told my husband.

"Then quit your job," he said.

"We have lived on two incomes for so many years."

"How about this?" he said. "Let's plan toward you coming home a year from now. Take some time to think this through, and I'll try to pick up some extra work. Set the resignation date now."

With a definite plan and a projected stop date at work,

energy flowed through my veins. Walking around the block and shopping for fresh fruits and veggies became pleasurable treats, not drudgery. The journey to frugality boosted my self-esteem as I knew I had hope for a future. I found myself more productive at work and at home. I had one year to implement our plan. With the same vigor with which I had written business plans for the company, I charted our family's year-to-freedom strategy. Sacrifices were made to pay off debt while increasing our savings. We would downsize our lifestyle to reach our aspirations.

Older women offered their wisdom on how to manage a family on a shoestring. Mom taught me to plan menus from the grocery's weekly sale ads while maximizing nutrition. I studied how to serve home cooked meals that rivaled the best local restaurants for a fraction of the cost. Meredith learned to cook alongside her mom and grandmother for a dad who appreciated it all.

Shopping at yard sales and thrift stores became a regular Saturday morning game. A mother of five invited us along to teach me the rules and art of negotiation. I found it similar to bargaining for limited resources among departments at work. In fact, many of my executive training skills were transferable to home management. It seemed that corporate lessons played well on the home front.

During that year-to-freedom, my schedule was as busy as ever, with the added pressure of achieving our family goal. Yet we remained optimistic, hopeful, and positive. Creativity reigned as we discovered ways to orient our lives toward our purpose. I had more energy, slept better, ditched the migraines, and experienced less anxiety. Everyone relaxed as we embraced a planned future together.

For me, the myth of health and happiness as a full-time executive and full-time mom was like serving two masters. Both wanted all my attention. I fell in love with home and became frustrated with my corporate career. Ten years later, I combine part-time work and home into a satisfying combo. However, at that stressful time in my life, the decision to choose one master took me off the rocky road to illness and put me on the highway of hope and health.

— Marylane Wade Koch —

Mind Over Matter

"I'm forty-eight," I whined to my friend Ilene, "but I feel like I'm eighty-four."

"But you look great," my friend responded. "I can't see a single wrinkle on your face."

Thanks to some heavy-duty moisturizer and well-placed make-up, that statement may have been true. However, what appeared at skin level was much different than what I felt taking hold beneath the surface—arthritis. The aches and pains first came upon me slowly in my early forties. In the years that followed, I never let my stiff fingers, creaky knees, or sore shoulders slow me down. Yet when the malady settled in my lower back, further aggravating on old injury, I had no choice but to take notice.

The constant ache in my back followed me everywhere I went like an unwelcome companion. Walking, sitting, bending, even lying in bed was, at best, uncomfortable most of the time. I dreaded getting in and out of my car thanks to the stabbing pains that radiated through my hips each time I shifted my weight. After seeing a movie, I needed to take a few bobbling steps before my regular gait returned and I could safely exit the theater. Even lifting myself from the sofa after watching just a few minutes of television required an equal amount of stretching before I was limber enough to walk into the kitchen for a snack.

Once fiercely self-reliant and above-average active, I found myself suddenly avoiding the most mundane of movements, using "my back" as an excuse. Replace that burned-out light bulb? Well, I would... but my back. Weed the garden? Not since my back started aching. Lift and carry those supermarket bags? You guessed it. No can do, thanks to my back.

One day, I bent over as I towel-dried my hair—and got stuck. What felt like an electric shock ran through my left hip, down the back of my leg, into the arch of my foot and stayed with me for a full ten minutes. Tears came to my eyes. The pain was so powerful that I couldn't even open my mouth to call out to my husband for help. The next morning, in a slightly reduced state of agony, I visited my doctor.

"Sciatica," he told me, "brought on by complications of injury, arthritis, and general weakness of the back muscles." He sent me off with the name of an over-the-counter pain reliever, a pamphlet outlining some helpful back exercises, and the recommendation to walk at least one mile each day. I followed his advice and the sciatica did subside. Yet that original nagging discomfort in my back stayed with me.

Back pain soon became my number one topic of conversation and I quickly found several other sufferers all too willing to commiserate over our poor fortune. As the old saying goes, misery loves company, and several of us would meet regularly to discuss our diagnoses and failed treatments. We were a beat-up, broken-down bunch of gals to be sure, grimacing at each step we took, a collective moan resounding as we took our seats. One woman wore a neck brace. Another regularly used a walker. Yet another arrived wheelchair bound.

When I returned home after one such meeting, I took a good look at my own reflection: hunched and limping. There, in front of that mirror, I laid it on the line. "God willing, you've got between thirty and forty years left on this earth," I said. "If you don't pull yourself together this situation will only get worse. Do you really want to give up? Already?"

"No!" I answered, stomping my foot for emphasis. "I might have pain, but I will not let pain have me."

From that day forward, I made every effort to stand straight, to walk strong, to stop wincing at each twist or turn, and especially to stop using "my back" as an excuse to not live my life as I should. In short, I no longer gave myself permission to baby my body. Even though the ache was still with me, it felt good to be back on my own two feet, so to speak. I became more active, and the more active I became, the happier I felt. And the happier I felt, the less I noticed the pain. In fact, by the time my next support group meeting arrived, I realized that I was pain-free and had been for several weeks. That afternoon, when it was my turn to speak, I announced that after many years I found myself feeling well. The next time I attended the meeting, still pain-free, I admitted shyly that I believed I had experienced a miracle.

Now, a full year after my "miracle," I have resumed all my normal activities. I walk, bicycle, and swim. And when I go to the movies, I get up out of my seat swiftly, shake off any stiffness and exit without fanfare. I have shoveled snow in the winter, pulled weeds in the summer, danced at a wedding in the spring, and raked leaves in the fall. Of course, I continue with my doctor's prescribed regimen of exercise and do remain cautious about certain movements he does not recommend. Yet, I attribute my newfound feeling of wellness to my change in attitude. Now, when a pinch or pull threatens to settle in my body, I no longer give in. Instead, I think back to the conversation that took place in front of my mirror, stamp my foot, and simply say, "No!"

— Monica A. Andermann —

Your Mind and Your Body: Best Friends for Life

Introduction

Best friends are tight. They have common interests. They share similar goals. They spend a lot of time together. They usually know where the other is. If their relationship hits rough waters, best friends batten down the hatches and weather the storm. They identify what the relationship needs and work toward finding their groove again. For great health, your mind and body need to be best friends. It's up to you to make sure the relationship is a strong one you can both count on.

Mention of the classic mind and body connection problem is a good place to start a discussion about how thoughts and feelings are linked to your physical health. Just how are the mind and body connected? How do they communicate? They are connected somehow, right? Never has such a special relationship between two things been so logical, yet so mysterious. Philosophers, scientists, and theologians have hammered on this mind-numbing question for centuries, only to agree that there's so much more to understand.

Throughout the following pages, I'll be sharing information

from contemporary research, my clinical experiences with courageous patients, and my thoughts gleaned from my own first-hand experiences with thinking and health. Experience is truly one of the best teachers. It certainly has been in my case.

Your Body Is a Tattletale

Several years ago, a physician friend asked me to join his efforts on a trip to work with homeless street kids in La Paz, Bolivia. For years he had developed relationships and found ways of connecting with parentless children who were facing some of life's grimmest circumstances. He thought the timing was right to bring a psychologist into the fold to help train the service workers in the area. I journeyed with a group to Bolivia, where we worked in the city as well as traveled to remote areas, visiting orphanages and churches, which commonly became the homes of children abandoned by their parents.

Though I provided much needed education and psychological intervention to Bolivian counselors, laypeople and pastors, the toughest job was being on the streets with the kids. We offered them support, understanding, and, at bare minimum, a human connection with someone who genuinely cared about them. The children were living in horrific squalor in alleys, in sewage drains, in cardboard shanties. They were seen as social nuisances, the equivalent of human rats. Many of them had physical injuries sustained from living on the streets. Gashes caused by glass and garbage covered their bare feet. Cuts and bruises sustained from fighting one another for food defiled the kids' bodies, while infection was common because antiseptics and antibiotics were not available to them.

The throbbing psychological and physical pain these kids endured was conveniently soothed by huffing inhalants from small wads of cloth. The inhalant high would give them warmth at night, and cool both their emotions and hunger pangs during the day.

My physician friend filled a healthcare void with an extraordinarily challenging medical specialty: helping street kids whose diet consisted of leftovers salvaged from garbage cans, food offered in exchange for prostitution, and the occasional special treat of a fried chicken head on a stick from a rare benevolent cart vendor. I left Bolivia with these images burned in my mind, wondering how effective I'd really been in making a dent in such a pervasive, hardly comprehensible problem.

I had been back in the United States about a month when I started developing some unpleasant gastrointestinal symptoms. I tried managing them with over-the-counter remedies, but eventually met with my primary care physician. Having traveled to a third world country, there was some concern that I had an atypical bacterial infection. If I did, it was turning out to be tougher than any run-of-the-mill stomach bug swimming in unsanitary water. After a series of tests, including my inaugural colonoscopy that turned up nothing, the specialist started me on a series of potent medications. When one didn't work, he'd try another.

One day, after several months of a disrupted lifestyle and a hovering diagnosis of irritable bowel syndrome, my pharmacist told me I was out of prescription benefits for the year and would now have to pay over four hundred dollars a month for my medications. That expense, remember, was for medication that wasn't working. I was enraged. It was at that very moment, a moment I still remember vividly years later, that I told the pharmacist I wasn't going to pay for the medicine and to put it back on her shelf. In fact, I brazenly told her I didn't even need the medicine anymore. As I spoke those words, I began to engage my brain in my own healing process. My mind and my body were starting to regroup for the first time since I'd been to Bolivia.

You see, I had been chasing a medical problem that should have been addressed psychologically. The way my body and brain connected was a lot like Deborah Ellis's friend Sue whose body became rigid and hot at the mere thought of money. Once I started talking more about my negative emotions, my physical symptoms started to subside, and my body began to heal. I had suppressed my feelings of hopelessness and anger about the injustices I had witnessed in Boliva, wrapped it up in a nice package and put it away. I thought I was done with the third-world experience, but my body told me otherwise. That trip to the pharmacy allowed me to access my anger—an anger I had stifled since witnessing the horrifying lives of the street kids of La Paz. Who was I kidding? Psychologists' lives are stressful already. Add to that a firsthand experience of seeing those who can't protect themselves living in such inhumane conditions. No doubt, I suppressed the anger—shelved it you might say—and hadn't done anything about it. As a result, my body tattled on my mind.

Through that experience I learned to talk about stress in a different way. I'd thought psychologists were supposed to keep their emotions and coping strategies in order. Well, I've come a long way since then, and as result of solid research and personal experience I'll be sharing the handy theory of cognitive behavioral psychology with you. Cognitive behavioral psychology is the key to my understanding of how the mind and body connect. It can be a key for you, too.

Brainpower Can Fuel Healing

Throughout my career, I've been surrounded by gifted physicians and healthcare professionals who have gone beyond the call of duty to tackle maladies with great success. I believe most of those miracle workers, however, would agree that brainpower is an indispensable part of maintaining great health. Brainpower can fuel healing. How you think can directly affect how you feel. Please don't misunderstand. I'm not trying to convince you that every ailment you have is in your head. Many diagnoses are far from that, in fact. If you have any medical concerns, you should always see your healthcare provider. Whether you are trying to maintain good health or trying to restore it, you need to include your brain in the process.

As I mentioned before, one of the trickiest brainteasers of all time remains: How do the brain and body really connect? We are each uniquely biologically and neurologically wired. Ancient philosophers like Plato, Aristotle, and Descartes knew some connection must exist, but couldn't put a fine bead on it. Even with advancing biomedical sciences and technology, we still know little about how the mind-body connection exactly works, but that's not to say we don't have a few strong leads.

Functional magnetic resonance imaging (fMRI) has allowed researchers to scan the human brain (along with many other parts of the human anatomy) to actually see how it's being used by its owner. Think of an fMRI as a colorful three-dimensional X-ray of your brain on a computer screen that shows when, where, and how your brain changes during different types of activities. Thanks to fMRI studies, doctors and researchers can estimate more accurately how the brain works under a variety of conditions. But we need to put a twist on the ancient mind-body conundrum. Rather than wondering about how it exists, we must embrace the mystery of the connection and start engaging our brains to better take charge of our health. Don't worry if you're not a biology person. You don't have to be. Don't be concerned if you never took a chemistry class or don't know what the periodic table is. You don't need to know. You've stepped onto an airplane without understanding the physics of flight. You've marveled at a skyscraper without studying architecture. Just by being curious, you've positioned yourself to start learning about your brain and how it can positively affect your health.

One thing is for sure: you are an expert on yourself, including how you think, feel, behave, make decisions, and connect with others. And because you're an expert on yourself, you are poised to become the foremost authority on how your brain influences your personal health. In order to do this though, you need to understand what cognitive behavioral psychology is and how to start integrating it into your life.

Cognitive Behavioral Psychology: Build a Toolbox for Great Health

Cognitive behavioral psychology is the most examined psychological approach in the research literature and it can lead to permanent, positive change in the brain. In cognitive behavioral psychology's most simplistic terms, the "cognitive" part focuses on thinking and thought while the "behavioral" piece has to do with actions, new or old behaviors, habits, and sometimes, social interactions. The beauty of taking a cognitive behavioral therapy (CBT) approach comes from the connection between thought and behavior. CBT allows you to access the brain and start changing it. You can actually activate your own thoughts, use them in instructive and corrective ways, and change your behavior for the better. When you begin thinking in a healthy way, you'll probably start noticing changes in emotions and behaviors. As you read through the next few chapters, you will understand more about how your thinking affects behavior, particularly as it relates to improving or maintaining health.

An easy way to understand cognitive behavioral psychology is to use an ABC model. "A" represents what is referred to as the Activating event, such as a situation you are in or a set of circumstances facing you. The "B" represents Beliefs, which are the thoughts that you have in the moment of the activating event. For example, a patient I'll call Allison. Her activating event occurs when she walks into a large room full of people at an after-hours networking mixer. Her belief is that everyone in the room is staring at her and thinking negatively about her. Now, for the "C" in the model: It stands for Consequences, which are usually undesirable or uncomfortable emotions or behaviors that become a problem. As a result of Allison's belief that people are judging her harshly when she walks into the room, she experiences a high level of anxiety and quickly leaves the room.

In cognitive behavioral therapy, we take aim at the belief (the "B") so we can affect the consequence (the "C"). Take a look at the box below so you can see how I have mapped out the ABC model for Allison.

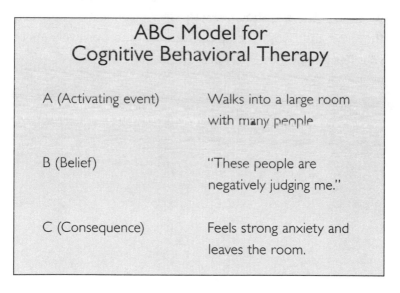

ABC Model for Cognitive Behavioral Therapy

A (Activating event)	Walks into a large room with many people
B (Belief)	"These people are negatively judging me."
C (Consequence)	Feels strong anxiety and leaves the room.

For Allison, it may be tough in the moment to understand how her beliefs are creating her anxiety. But as you look at the situation on paper, it's clear that the views she holds about herself and the situation are inaccurate. To help Allison identify her inaccuracies so she can change them, I'd point out that not everyone in the room is looking at her. Nor are all of the people in the room thinking the exact same thing about her. That would be humanly impossible. Inaccurate thoughts and beliefs are often described as irrational or distorted. I like to use the word "inaccurate" about "wrong" thinking because that means we can improve our accuracy about how we perceive ourselves and the world around us.

Whether you've heard of cognitive behavioral therapy before, or if this is a brand new idea for you, I'm glad you're interested in learning about how to use the connection between the mind and body to employ your brain to positively affect your health. You'll catch on quickly.

———

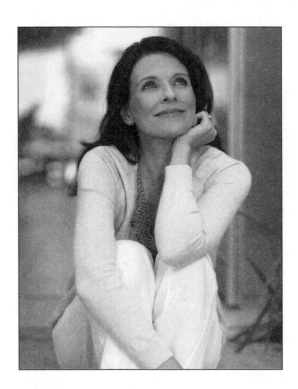

Chapter 2
The Brain Secrets that Healthy People Know

The Choice

Dr. Lee looked up at me after noting my chart: "Your blood pressure is elevated again. In fact, the reading is even higher than your last visit." He softened his gaze. "Is there anything going on in your life that would cause it to rise like this?"

"No," I mumbled, "nothing is going on." I closed my eyes and sighed. I just didn't feel like repeating the list of troubles I had been experiencing over the past year: my added responsibilities due to my father's failing health, that leaking roof that seemed to defy repair, or my problems at the office compounded by the threat of impending lay-offs.

After promising to remove all unnecessary sodium from my diet, my doctor gave me a one-month reprieve. If, at the end of one month's time, my blood pressure did not return to an acceptable range, he would prescribe medication. The thought of being reliant on pills at only middle age really bothered me, and I left his office determined to find a way to help my blood pressure return to normal.

As I pulled out of the parking lot and onto the road, I felt my face redden. Why were all the other drivers moving so slowly? Didn't they know I had to get to the supermarket before going to my dad's house to cook dinner for him? I huffed and puffed. Traffic was stop and go the whole way. Getting from Dad's house to mine afterward was no better and I griped to myself the entire trip. By the time I got to my own home and finished preparing dinner for my husband and me, the top of my head tingled. And when I went into my bedroom afterward with the intention of grabbing a magazine and relaxing, I found a pile of laundry waiting to be folded. My heart went into full-on palpitations. I flopped onto my bed and looked at my clock—it was already 10:30 p.m. No wonder I had high blood pressure.

That night, too wound-up to sleep, I sat in my kitchen nursing a cup of chamomile tea as I listened to a late-night radio talk show. The radio psychologist was taking phone calls and dispensing glib advice. Unhappy marriage? Dump your spouse. Disobedient children? Administer punishment. Life got you down? Just whistle a happy tune. Ugh. I reached for the plug, ready to rip it right out of the socket. Then a tiny, tired voice came on.

"I'm just so disgusted with my daily grind. I hate going to the supermarket. I hate cooking dinner. I hate doing laundry," the caller explained.

"Well, then get a maid," the radio psychologist said.

"I can't afford one," replied the caller. "I have three small children and I'm a stay-at-home mom."

"Listen honey," the radio psychologist started, "if you have three small children, you'll be going to the supermarket, cooking dinner, and doing laundry for a very long time. You can either be miserable when you do your chores, or you can slap a smile on your face when you do your chores. You decide."

I flicked off the radio. What did that fancy-schmancy talk-show psychologist know? Probably she had a maid to clean her house and a nanny for her children—if she even had any children at all. I went to bed, my heart bumping around my chest.

The next morning I was off and running again, grumbling the whole time. After work, I stomped into the pharmacy to pick up a prescription for my father. Behind the counter the pharmacist stood, phone in one hand, a stack of prescriptions in the other. When she saw me, she looked up and sent the most beautiful smile my way. "I'll be right with you, dear," she said in a voice that flowed like honey.

As I waited, I turned and noticed that a line had now formed. Behind me, two customers chatted. "The pharmacist here is always so busy," said one to the other, "but she never lets it get to her. Just look at that smile."

I thought about the talk-show psychologist's comments the night before and checked my own expression, eyes steeled toward the counter, lips down in a scowl. So when the pharmacist handed me my dad's medication and wished me a good day, I made a half-hearted attempt to smile back. "You have a good day, too," I answered, my eyes fixed firmly on the exit.

I still had one more errand to run that night before I could get home. Scrambling across the street, I made my way to the library to return a book. Another line. I shuffled from foot to foot. The patron at the head of the line was arguing with the clerk over a late fee. The clerk made a quick joke and the two women laughed. Then the patron paid the fee and left without fanfare. The next patron in line had at least ten books to return. The whole while, the clerk chatted with her pleasantly. Next, my turn. I placed my book on the counter. "On time," I mumbled, and turned to leave.

"You have a good evening," sang the clerk.

I turned back and looked at her. "Uh, you too," I said. Then, as though tugged by some nameless force, I returned to the counter. "You're just about the calmest, kindest person I've ever met," I blurted. "What's your secret?"

She looked across the counter at me and grinned. "No secret," she said. "It's just a choice."

A choice. Just like that radio psychologist said. It looked like the time had come for me to make a choice, too. I could go through life stomping and grumbling or I could smile and sing. From now on, I was going to opt for the latter.

It wasn't easy at first. In fact it was hard. My initial attempts at holding a sincere smile on my face felt a bit like wearing a Halloween mask. Yet when I found myself singing along to the car radio instead of cursing traffic, and humming as I did my housework, I knew I was making real progress. After a few weeks, I noticed that the strange tingling at the top of my head and those intermittent palpitations seemed to be gone. Not only that, I just felt better overall. Calmer. Happier. Life was no longer a burden, but something to be enjoyed.

At the end of the month, I returned to my doctor. This time he had good news: blood pressure normal. He noted his chart and looked up at me. "It looks like reducing your sodium intake really helped," he commented.

"Yep," I answered, a bright smile lighting my face, "it certainly did."

"Keep it up," he said, "and I'll see you next year."

"You bet," I sang out as I left. Then I looked back over my shoulder. "And Dr. Lee, you have a great day."

I knew I would.

— Monica A. Andermann —

Don't Stop...
Keep on Going!

The first time I met Monte, he was complaining about everybody celebrating his 99th birthday. It was hurting his chances for a date.

"No woman wants to go out with a 100-year-old man," he said with that infectious laugh. I often heard his laughter over the next few years in the church lobby where he ushered three services each Sunday morning. Celebrating his birthday didn't do too much damage to Monte's social life because I saw him out with two different ladies that next week. I learned that Monte loved people and enjoyed getting to know them.

I decided to interview Monte for the magazine where I am editor. Some of my interest in Monte stemmed from a nagging thought that I might be getting old. I had recently found myself in a room thinking, "What did I come in here for?" And my day involved looking for... glasses, keys, book, letter, address... well, you know. The interview with Monte was the first of three, the beginning of a friendship I will always value and a change in how I handle aging.

Monte was a chemist and advanced the efforts in World War II by keeping his Fort Worth plant open and running at high production during those years. He delivered meals on wheels up until he turned 100. One day as Monte drove away from church he had a small accident, dropping his car into a ditch. The policeman revoked Monte's driver's license, explaining that at his age he needed to retest. Not being able to drive can be a blow of discouragement for most of us. Driving seems to be a symbol of independence, especially for Monte who loved to go and do. However he didn't sit inside and feel sorry for himself. He didn't argue and drive anyway—breaking the law. He asked someone to drive him to take the test. His neighbor volunteered, thinking it to be a waste of time. Monte passed the written test with a score of 100 and the driving test with flying colors. He received his new driver's license and continued helping the "old" people.

I asked him for his secret to long life. He recommended lots of water, no over-eating, and learning new things.

"The main thing," Monte said, "is I don't stop. If I wake up with a pain, I just put one foot in front of the other and I get going. I keep on doing."

Most of that doing was volunteering in the community, in the church, in the neighborhood. Monte was interested in others and stayed busy.

On my last visit to his house, he was raking the yard and answered my question regarding his health.

"Well, I'm feeling quite well," he said. "Except this one knee is giving me a little pain. I'm not sure what's wrong with it."

"Monte," I said. "It could be that the knee is 100 years old."

"Well, yes," he laughed. "And it's about to be 101."

This is when I evaluated Monte's zest for life and willingness to serve others. As an author and editor, I find myself sitting far too much. After Monte passed away, another friend came my way, one I could serve the way Monte had served others. My knees have been hurting a great deal lately but "I just put one foot in front of the other and I get going. I keep on doing..." and I keep on learning. If I hear of a new technology, I try to learn as much as possible about how to use it.

Helping others... old people with knees that hurt... keeps me young. I try to swim every day possible. I have learned to play an instrument, and with a group of friends, visit nursing homes every week. Helping others has helped me.

I believe in finding a quality that I admire in the people I love and applying that quality to my own life. Then part of that person lives on through me. I believe Monte's motto—keep going and keep learning—has kept me from sitting myself into bad health and slow thinking.

Now if I can only find my keys, I'll be on my way to go help others.

~ Peggy Purser Freeman ~

Numbers Don't Lie

T he word leapt off the page and seared itself on my brain. The letter I was holding came from my HMO with the results of a blood glucose test. "You have pre-diabetes. People with pre-diabetes have a high risk of developing diabetes in the future," it said bluntly.

I sat up, senses alert. I felt scared and threatened, like when I was in junior high and the math teacher called on me for an answer I didn't know. I'll admit I was a little defensive, too. Didn't my HMO realize I was a healthy person? I exercised. I'd been in good health throughout my life. I was in my sixties and I had always eaten whatever I wanted.

But it was time to be honest with myself. My weight had crept up in the past decade. I wasn't exercising as much as I used to. And other numbers besides weight and blood glucose had edged upward: cholesterol, blood pressure, triglycerides. I might have been a poor math student, but I knew that numbers don't lie. I remember how I felt if I got a low grade on a test; reading the "pre-diabetes" letter produced similar feelings of humiliation.

Although my HMO was trying to slap the "pre-diabetic" label on me, I refused to buy into it. It would mean changing my eating and exercise habits.

Before I could change my habits I had to change my thinking.

I considered some assumptions I held about myself. We all have them—it's what we tell ourselves about ourselves. The messages, a mixture of positive and negative, shape our identity. They may have started in childhood and originated with parents, teachers, siblings and friends. But now they come from a quiet voice heard only by ourselves. Things like: You're bad at math. You're a good speller. You can't carry a tune. You're a good friend. You have a good sense of direction. You're a self-starter. You can't draw. You're a morning person.

I had always told myself I could eat whatever I wanted. When I was at a party or potluck, I tried every dish and then complimented the cook. I always cleaned my plate. I loved potatoes no matter how they were cooked.

Now I had to update those assumptions. I quit bragging that I could eat anything I wanted. That might have been true when I was younger, but it wasn't true anymore, not if I wanted to be healthy. I realized that I can't eat deep-fried foods and desserts every night. I can't eat as much cheese and butter as I'd like. I can't eat potato chips and other salty snacks.

But that sounded too negative, so I changed "can't" to "don't" and the messages I told myself became more convincing: I don't eat pie, bagels or donuts. I love potatoes, but I don't eat them every day. I don't eat a lot of meat. I don't eat creamy salad dressings. I don't drink sugary sodas. I don't eat at fast-food restaurants.

Not wanting to feel deprived, I focused on positive

assumptions: I want to be a healthy person. I eat healthy foods. I love fresh vegetables and fruit. I can eat brown rice and whole-grain bread as easily as white rice and bread. I prefer home-cooked meals made from fresh ingredients to restaurant food or prepared foods.

After weeks of consciously repeating those sentences like a mantra, I started believing them. In a way, I began to change my identity. Then the good habits fell into place easily.

Now I eat more vegetarian dishes. At a restaurant, I usually order fish and salad. Or if I have Mexican food or pasta, I take half of it home. I no longer feel obligated to sample all of the goodies at a party—I can let someone else take over that role. Instead of cleaning my plate at dinner, I often save part for lunch the next day. When I see tempting, fat-ridden foods in TV commercials I tell myself, "I'll eat that again someday, but not today or tomorrow."

Since my husband is the cook in our house, I convinced him to make some changes. Now he reaches for olive oil more often than butter when he's cooking. He switched to whole-grain pasta and low-sodium products. We no longer keep ice cream and cookies on hand but save them for special occasions.

We relish our high-quality, plant-based diet. Tomatoes, spinach, blueberries, avocados, pears, mushrooms, zucchini, eggplant—our market offers a wealth of healthy and yummy produce that can be turned into fabulous meals.

Eating well is a primary pleasure, but life doesn't have to be all about food. Instead of just looking forward to my next meal,

I focus on other pleasurable pursuits: photography, reading, working puzzles, finding new music for my MP3 player—and physical activities too.

The "pre-diabetes" letter said, "Even a small amount of weight loss by healthy eating and increased physical activity can lower your risk of developing diabetes up to 60 percent." Now there's a number I like.

Rejecting the "pre-diabetes" label, I chose some new labels for myself. Now, I'm an avid walker. In the summer, I'm a swimmer. At least once a week I'm a biker and sometimes I'm a hiker.

Best of all, a year after receiving the letter, I'm no longer a pre-diabetic. When I went for my last checkup, my blood glucose was well within the normal range, and so was my blood pressure. Total cholesterol was down by 10 points, and triglycerides were down almost 40 points.

Another number is the one that lights up when I step onto the scale. A year ago it was 152 and now it reads 138. Being healthy was my primary goal, not losing weight. But slimming down is a side benefit I will gladly accept.

Maybe there's another assumption I should update—the one that says I'm bad at math. Now I feel proud of my healthy lifestyle, the way I felt in school when I did well on a test. Numbers don't lie, and I've made them work in my favor.

~ Kathryn Wilkens ~

Exercise
Can Be Fun
at Any Age

When I turned fifty nearly three years ago, I vowed that I would change the way I looked and felt. I had recently gone through cancer surgery and treatments and was feeling better. Yet, I struggled with my diabetes, my weight, my energy level, and then my blood pressure.

As a full-time writer and someone who was never really "into" athletics, I figured that my only hope was dieting, and that I wouldn't try the exercise part. Where would I find the time? The energy? The interest?

Like most people, I tried a variety of known and self-imposed diets. Some worked for a while, but it was too easy to revert to old eating habits.

When a friend told me she was beginning to walk for exercise, I thought that I might try it. So, every once in a while, whenever I felt like getting out and doing it (which wasn't very often), I'd walk around a local shopping center or at the dog park. It was good, but sporadic.

Suddenly, my friend began telling me how she was walking one, then two, then three miles a day. She was losing weight and feeling wonderful. Then she was going to the gym and walking and working out on the machines. It all sounded difficult, but I was proud of her.

When she began reporting on her astounding weight loss and how her blood sugar levels were staying in a normal range, I decided it was time to make my own commitment. I gave myself a challenge to keep up with her.

The summer of 2011 was a tough one in Texas. Weeks and months of over 100-degree temperatures every day. So I became an ardent morning mall walker. I began with 20 minutes at a leisurely pace. It wasn't long before I was walking faster, pushing myself. Then, the walks were 30 minutes and soon 45. At my pace, I knew I had to be walking two miles at a time.

My husband, a teacher, saw how the walks were giving me more energy, lowering my weight, and even more importantly, my blood sugar. Although he gardened those summer mornings, he was encouraged to walk with me in the evenings. I began walking twice a day, two miles at a time.

The weight didn't just fall off, but I could see a difference on the scale and on my blood sugar readings every day.

When friends invited us to swim in their pool whenever they were swimming, we began spending two or three nights a week at the pool instead of walking. I continued my morning walks. But I discovered that swimming, not just floating around, was relaxing, refreshing, and even more athletic than walking. I was hooked on the combination.

My best friend from college was impressed with my commitment. She had always been a walker, but decided to try the pool at her housing association as well. Soon, she was swimming laps every morning and reporting them to me. I was reporting my exercise to an online friend who had encouraged me in the beginning. My husband followed in my footsteps.

When our teacher friends went back to work and no longer had much time for the pool, and my husband wasn't walking with me at the mall, I discovered that our local community center had both an indoor pool and an exercise machine room.

Now, I am excited every day to begin my mornings with God, then working on my writing, then off to the community center to walk one to three miles on the treadmill or bike on the bicycle machine before jumping into the wonderfully refreshing pool to swim laps for thirty minutes.

I'm amazed at how I, an un-athletic person who waited until her fifties to begin an exercise routine, have stuck to it. I am thoroughly enjoying every minute of it.

I am blessed by the friend who began this routine in her own life. I pray that I will see the wonderful results she has in my own weight loss. But if not, I know that at least I've gotten my body active for the first time in many years, and I lowering both my blood sugar and blood pressure.

Who knew exercise at fifty could be so much fun?

~ Kathryn Lay ~

The Brain Secrets that Healthy People Know

Introduction

It is fascinating to watch a documentary about how something complex is assembled, to read a biography of an interesting person, or sneak a behind-the-scenes look into a favorite movie or television show. Watching the gag reel of outtakes or the making of a movie can be just as entertaining as the movie itself. It is human nature to desire insight into the inner workings of something. And, it's simply amazing when reality is revealed from a different perspective. One of my favorite such experiences occurred when I was co-authoring a Harvard Medical School book called *The Winner's Brain*.

My colleagues and I had the rare opportunity to visit the set of *Sesame Street* at Kaufman Astoria Studios in Queens, New York. As guests of Kevin Clash, the unmistakable voice behind and gifted hands inside the always endearing Elmo, we sat in tall director's chairs just steps from Oscar's trashcan and the iconic green signpost. We watched as talented puppeteers gave life to some of children's (and adults') favorite friends. Even if it's been years since you've watched *Sesame Street*, I'm confident you recall it well and experience a fair amount of nostalgia as a result. Seeing *Sesame Street* from the outside on television gives a one-dimensional perspective, but being in the studio—on the inside—offers a different viewpoint about how skill, creativity, and ability complexly meld together to make something involved seem so routine.

Your brain is much the same way. On the outside it appears life moves along without much thought. However, behind the scenes your brain has special, unique ways of handling situations. Simple, practical phenomena occur, many of which healthy people recognize and use regularly. I want to get you up to speed on some "brain secrets," if you will, particularly in areas that you need to master so you can start using your thinking to enhance and strengthen your health positively.

Four Secrets for Healthy Thinking

Secret #1: Fire Dr. Google and Get Some Closure
Healthy people get accurate information in legitimate ways, and then use the information to their advantage. I can't count the number of times I have seen someone in my office who has been searching the Internet, Googling symptoms and self-diagnosing. Even more, I can't ever remember a time someone was satisfied with any answer they found about their health from Dr. Google, or anywhere else on the Internet for that matter.

The human brain naturally tracks toward closure and that's why people search incessantly for information. Closure is a foundational concept in the theory of Gestalt therapy. Gestalt therapy is a multidimensional, cognitive based therapy that emphasizes self-regulation in particular life circumstances. Closure is like the last and final piece of an individual's life experience puzzle that allows an event or story to make sense and conclude. In short, closure happens when a process or an event is completed.

Think about how closure plays a role in these situations: You probably don't like it if you are told the set-up of a joke but then the punch line isn't delivered. You're dissatisfied at the end of a season finale episode if it leaves you hanging until the next season. And you can rarely stop trying to think of someone's name or a fact that you have forgotten. Since you are missing important information, closure hasn't happened, and you are bothered emotionally.

When critical information about your health is missing, you're apt to search for it, too. But chasing information about symptoms on blogs and websites, or in threads and in social media, usually leads to increased anxiety. Why? Closure isn't happening. You aren't finding a clear, satisfactory answer to your health question and the likelihood that you actually will is quite low. Reading information from such outlets will typically increase anxiety rather than alleviate it, as well as increase the need for even more closure because further potential health "problems" are uncovered or self-diagnosed. If scouring the Internet is simply too tempting, then try to focus exclusively on educating yourself about what your doctor has diagnosed and recommended as a sound, research-based treatment for you.

You can and should use reliable information to reinforce getting better and staying healthy. If you'd like, ask your doctor which reputable sources are the best for information that aligns with his or her treatment recommendations.

Secret #2: Recognize and Eliminate
Unhealthy Defense Mechanisms

Healthy people refuse to play mind games with themselves. Although it would be rare today to find someone practicing Sigmund Freud's exact brand of psychology, you will still find many therapists utilizing his concepts. Freud defined a group of behaviors and ways of acting he called defense mechanisms. Defense mechanisms do exactly what they sound like they do. They protect us from negative feelings or uncomfortable emotions and ideas. From my experience, healthy people are able to recognize two significant defense mechanisms and use them to their advantage rather than allow them to pose as stumbling blocks impeding healthy thinking. Although Freud's menu of defense mechanisms is vast, you won't need to know all of them. Just focus on the following two so you can make healthy psychological steps toward feeling great.

The first defense mechanism is a classic one: Denial. For the most part, denial and healthy thinking simply do not mix. In some cases, denial can actually be healthy in small doses. It can give you some space and time to develop a plan of response or adjust to a new, stressful circumstance. In the long run, however, if you are going to maintain a healthy lifestyle, you have to not let this defense mechanism get the best of you. As long as you use denial over extended periods of time, you are putting yourself at risk. If not recognized and navigated, denial can be the single barrier standing between you and healthy living. It may be difficult to admit you need to change behaviors so you can live a healthier lifestyle.

Take, for instance, a man I'll call Jack. He's an obese man who was told by his physician that he must lose 50 pounds to reduce the risk of a heart attack. Jack later told his wife that his doctor seemed inexperienced and probably doled out boilerplate recommendations to him like he does to his other patients. This is an example of denial. Despite having objective information about his weight, Jack did not accept that a problem exists and may eventually experience cardiac complications that may cost him his life.

Another defense mechanism that often buttresses denial is rationalization. Rationalization occurs when you make up excuses (usually very good ones, in fact) to justify your behaviors. Somewhere down deep you know that your behaviors are unhealthy or are in need of adjustment, but you want to keep doing them for some reason—often for pleasure or escape. When you rationalize, you create reasons why unhealthy behaviors are okay or why change is unnecessary. Perhaps you have heard a smoker say about his smoking, "We all have to die sometime." While it's a ridiculously poor excuse, this statement is a perfect example of rationalization. Again, it may be difficult to admit you need to change behaviors so you can improve the quality of your thinking, but healthy people do it anyway.

Secret # 3: Learn How Change Happens
Healthy people learn to change and adapt. I keep a collection

of jokes about psychologists and one of my favorites poses the question, "How many psychologists does it take to change a light bulb?" The answer is, "Only one, but the light bulb has to want to change."

In my work with patients who want to change, I suggest they think of change being like a dimmer switch, rather than a light switch, because change occurs gradually, not immediately. When it becomes necessary for us to change behaviors, it seems the pressure to change can be felt almost instantly. Just like Kathryn Lay who had undergone cancer treatments and wanted to improve her life, you may have a medical event, get disheartening test results, or a close friend or relative who reminds you of yourself dies. But, change doesn't work in an instant. It takes time, so be prepared.

James Prochaska, Ph.D., professor at the University of Rhode Island, has dedicated his career to understanding how behavioral change occurs. His well-respected theories are incredibly useful when developing strategies to become healthier. From the previous example about rationalization, you'll recall that Dr. Isaac delivered the news to Jack that he needed to lose weight. Obviously, Jack wouldn't lose the weight by the next day. But if Jack knew Prochaska's stages of change, he could start the process right away. Healthy people seem to understand how to change and are patient as they slowly work toward better health. Below is a brief description of Prochaska's stages of change. If you are in the process of change, or perhaps need to consider making a change, read through the stages and see where in the process you might be. By understanding how change occurs, you can think more positively about how to promote a healthy lifestyle.

Prochaska's Stages of Change

Stage 1: Pre-contemplation

Individuals in the pre-contemplation stage of change are not even aware that change needs to occur in their lives. At this point, someone like your doctor may tell you that you need to make a change. If you think it's possible that you could be in the pre-contemplation stage, begin seriously thinking about the behaviors that might need modification. Try considering fully what life would be like if you made any change, even a small one. And if you are certain that you don't need to make a change in spite of being asked to consider it by professionals, you may want to consider reading the section on healthy and unhealthy denial again.

Stage 2: Contemplation

In the contemplation stage, individuals have come to terms with the fact that change may indeed apply to them. However, they still remain ambivalent about change and haven't clearly made the decision to move toward it. If you find yourself in this category, it is okay if you have not committed to change. You may however want to try developing a pros and cons list and also remind yourself that you alone can make the decision to change. Information gathering can be an important strategy too—but not with Dr. Google! Be careful though, rationalization can easily rear its ugly head during this stage and talk you out of your best intentions to do something different.

Stage 3: Preparation

In the preparation stage, individuals are gearing up to face the work that is required to do something different. It is here that you may want to consider building social supports, strategically collaborating with a healthcare professional and working on any new skills that you'll need when you formally begin the change process.

Stage 4: Action

Once individuals have made a decision to change and geared up for the process, it's time to put the ball into play. Lasting anywhere from three to six months, the action stage allows for a transformation in behaviors to take root. Although the behavior has not yet become permanent, the action stage gives you the opportunity to become more familiar with it and work out the kinks through practice. Those people in the action stage may benefit from trying to predict and plan for obstacles that get in the way of behavior change. You can practice telling yourself that the new behavior is actually part of who you are, and also make sure you stay well connected to social supports.

Stage 5: Maintenance

People in the maintenance stage of change are in the home stretch and have worked hard practicing new behaviors over the last three to six months. This part of the process should include a constant commitment to the new behavior and lifestyle, making certain to reinforce it by noticing internal rewards and getting plenty of external rewards. Internal rewards are those factors that you experience psychologically. Joy, increased self-esteem, robust confidence and rejuvenated hope are all great examples of internal rewards that can motivate change. External rewards, on the other hand, are those factors that provide a more immediate payoff and keep you moving toward the goal. A size-smaller outfit, a relaxing massage, or a favorite latte at the corner coffee shop can serve as excellent external rewards for positive behavior change.

You can also bolster gains by predicting and eliminating triggers, those forces that could cause a relapse into old habits. Triggers can be places, people, emotions, situations, or memories, to name a few. If you do happen to relapse, don't panic. Those who relapse typically return to an earlier stage of change and start cycling from that point again.

Secret #4: The Red Flag of Discomfort

Healthy people have learned to tune into a particular type of anxiety that informs them when a positive healthy decision needs to be made. All of us have found ourselves in situations where we want to do something, but we know it is probably not good for us. Smokers undeniably know that smoking can lead to a variety of terminal illnesses, but they crave the next cigarette and still choose to smoke it—even if they have to stand in the rain or freezing temperatures. People with unhealthy eating habits know that irresponsible eating can lead to a myriad of health problems such as obesity or diabetes. To think in a healthy way, you can benefit from paying attention to the noticeable anxiety that occurs when you want to do something, but know it is not good for you.

In the late 1950s, theorist Leon Festinger developed the concept of cognitive dissonance. Cognitive dissonance occurs when you try to hold two conflicting ideas at once. As a result, anxiety or discomfort is experienced. Take Jennifer, for instance. She has a pining for cigarettes and at the same time the desire to be healthy. These desires are in conflict; thus, a noticeable feeling of discomfort or tension arises in her. This discomfort should serve as a red flag for Jennifer that a critical healthy decision needs to be made. A few paragraphs earlier we talked about rationalization. Beware: rationalization is usually employed to reduce the discomfort that results from conflicting ideas so you can do that which is more pleasurable. Remember the excuse that smokers "have to die sometime"? That is rationalization in action, to reduce discomfort between the two opposing ideas.

Healthy people recognize the red flag of discomfort, start watching for rationalizations, and then purposefully (and sometimes painfully) make the right choice. You too can recognize anxiety related to conflicting ideas and make a great choice, especially when your life or health is at risk now or in the future.

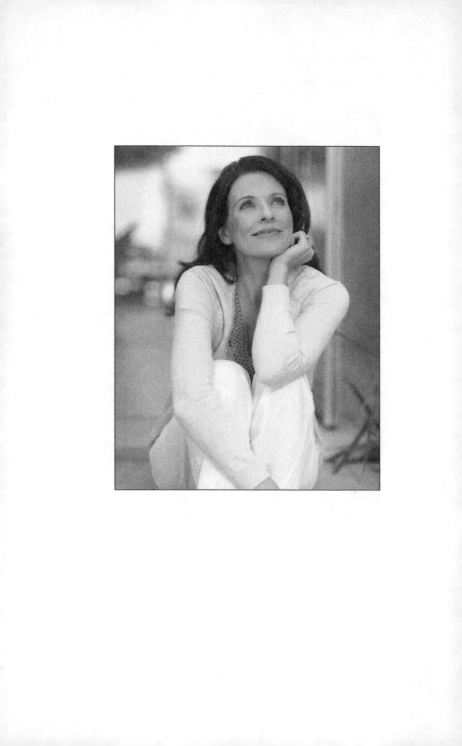

Chapter 3
Hope for the Best and *Expect* the Best

Open Heart

I t was a quiet room, sophisticated, but not ostentatious. The soothing decor was all there: a flat screen TV on the wall playing muted cartoons, the fish tank in the corner gurgling sleepily. A little boy squirmed on the couch nearby, his father hushing him distractedly. Assorted issues of *Better Homes and Gardens* lay strewn across the end table.

"Kristen?" came a pleasant voice from the office. "We're ready for you; come on back." That was me, the impatient teenager getting up from the couch near the child. I followed the pleasant woman to an exam room, an upscale closet with a high-tech examining table and chocolate-colored walls bedecked with diagrams of the heart. My father, taking a look at the examining table, commented it probably cost over $10,000. I made a note to look into cardiology as a possible career. Suddenly the door opened and an amicable nurse arrived to ask a few questions.

"So why are you coming to see the doctor today?"

I twitched with irritation. Why did she think I had come to the doctor today? Because I was just itching to experience my umpteenth doctor appointment in the last four months? But I checked myself and explained to the nurse that I was a competitive swimmer, that for a while I had been having trouble breathing at practice, that a dozen doctor's appointments had finally turned up a heart murmur that had somehow escaped everyone's notice for sixteen years. I calmly informed her that I had been sent to have an echocardiogram, an ultrasound of my heart, and I was here to receive the results of the test. She nodded her understanding and continued her questionnaire.

I didn't have time for this. I had homework and friends and swim team and a thousand other things more important than this appointment. Besides, I had done my research—most heart murmurs are benign, meaning they don't indicate any problem with the heart. I was an accomplished athlete. I knew there was nothing wrong with my heart.

A brief knock, then the cardiologist entered. A short, rather wide man of Indian descent, he had a squashed nose and warm brown eyes. Though balding, his hair retained a touch of color. He greeted us smiling, but something about that smile betrayed a hint of worry.

"I have just looked at the echocardiogram." He hesitated. He spoke in a thick accent. "I have just looked at the echocardiogram and it is not good news."

I felt my father's eyes upon me, though I did not return his glance.

The doctor continued. "It appears the right side of your heart is larger than the left. By 22 percent." He went on to explain that he saw two possible culprits—both congenital heart defects. The more likely, it seemed to him, was partial anomalous pulmonary venous return (PAPVR), which meant some of the veins leading from the lungs to the heart were not properly formed. This would require heart surgery, and soon. There was another option, though, an atrial septal defect (ASD), or a hole in the wall between the sides of my heart. Although the solution to this was also surgery, it would not involve cutting open my chest. A new procedure for this defect had been devised, one that involved inserting a catheter into a vein in the patient's leg and threading a sort of plug into the hole.

"But first I am sending you to a pediatric cardiologist for a definite diagnosis. He will know more about congenital defects. Now let me check availability...."

I had stopped listening. There was some mistake; there had to be. Walking back out past the serene waiting room, I turned and stole a glance, yearning for those moments just a half hour before. The fish, the TV humming silently, all was just as I had left it, but I was anything but the same. I realized I would be seeing a lot of this place.

I walked in silence back to the cars with my father. As he had come from work and I from school, we had driven separately. Now he opened the passenger door, sat down in my car beside me, and began to cry. I didn't know what to do, what to say, what to think. All I could feel was numb.

It was Thursday, January 6, 2011. The next week was the longest of my life. Explaining to my mother what had transpired, telling my friends, doing homework, eating, sleeping, thinking, thinking, thinking. I had been banned from swimming; all I could do was think.

Finally the day arrived for me to see the pediatric cardiologist. This time my father picked me up from school. Our conversation in the car was empty, shallow. It was just to fill the space.

We were greeted in the hospital by another cheery nurse—and another echocardiogram. I lay on the table for almost an hour, inundated by a familiar antiseptic smell, tortured by what-ifs. When I at last was released, I looked into the doctor's shadowed face, trying to anticipate the result. His expression was inscrutable. He turned away and, without looking at me, instructed me to dress and meet him in the exam room. My stomach turned. I changed quickly and came to the door. I paused for only a moment, then pushed it open.

This doctor was balding, with gray hair and goatee. His smile, though it lacked the natural warmth of my other doctor, was not without kindness.

He opened a small booklet. "Here's what you have," he said, pointing to the page describing the ASD—the hole, the catheterization procedure. He went on to explain all the details, but all I could feel was relief. Warm, glowing relief flooded my body, washing from my head to my toes. No painful surgery. No scar. I was sixteen. I would get to stay that way.

It wasn't until we were approaching the car that I was struck by the peculiarity of the situation. I had just found out I had a hole in my heart, and one would think I had been spared the death penalty. But, I realized, it was true. I was lucky.

Of course, I had always known I was fortunate. But never before had it hit home like this. What if it had been something more serious? What if my parents didn't have jobs and health care and couldn't afford the procedure? What if I didn't have such devoted parents? There are kids who don't make it to sixteen. There are kids who die as children, the hapless casualties of sickness, hunger, war, abuse, and neglect. Who am I to be worried about a scar? I am so lucky; I always have been.

On February 22, 2011, I underwent a procedure to close the hole in my heart. All went well. Since then I have read the booklet the pediatric cardiologist gave me cover to cover, and I am considering going into cardiology after all. Who knows? Maybe I can share a piece of my luck with the world.

— Kristen Finney, age 18 —

Brain, Body, and Beat

When my husband Bill and I started dance lessons seventeen years ago, I didn't expect dancing to transform my life. I wasn't even sure I'd be any good at it. But Bill wanted to dance, and we could do the activity together, so I was willing to try. At least Bill had experience to fall back on. When he was twelve, he learned to dance at the Cotillion Club at Ball State University in Muncie, Indiana, his hometown. He remembered the fun he had then and during the adult education classes he took later. My experience was limited to a few basic swing steps Bill had taught me when we dated. After our wedding, a decade passed before we signed up for lessons. By then we were in our forties, our lives filled with busy work schedules and community service commitments.

Had anyone suggested I would develop a passion for dancing, I would have said, "No way!" I did not perceive myself as a graceful or coordinated individual, although my favorite childhood activities did include roller skating and whirling hula hoops. As an adult, I stayed in shape through a hodgepodge of not-very-motivating exercises. My history of a rare tumor disorder and surgeries did little to boost my confidence regarding physical pursuits. I also feared my longtime hearing loss would prevent me from staying on beat.

Determined, and not one to shy away from challenging tasks, I signed up for group classes, private lessons, and social events. Dancing gave me a break from school social work, a job I found both satisfying and taxing. Away from work, I stepped into another world, one that relied less on thinking and more on movement. This shift allowed me to return refreshed for my job the next day.

Soon fitness benefits surfaced: increased stamina, improved posture, and better balance. "You look like a dancer!" others observed. New friendships expanded my circle of support. While I expected physical and social benefits, the rigor of dancing surprised me.

Learning new dances and advanced steps involved more skills than I had imagined. Dancing meant interpreting the music, executing step patterns and variations, making decisions, and responding quickly. Following a partner's lead requires split-second decisions. Leading involves choosing steps, patterns, and variations, and using floor space accurately. Both partners must cooperate to keep the beat of the music, and to interpret and integrate the style of the dance and mood of the music. Changing partners—giving and responding to leads with less familiar partners—helps dancers stay sharp.

Pursuing this passion outside work allowed me to focus better on the job. By engaging more completely with my daily tasks, I worried less about past situations or potential problems in the future. I approached unfamiliar situations with an increased ability to "think on my feet" and generate a variety of solutions.

When I slipped into dance shoes and began moving to music, my mind, body, and spirit felt connected, not only in dancing, but throughout my life. I dropped activities that no longer captured my interest. Dancing built my fitness and confidence on multiple levels, allowing me to more fully live with hearing loss, ongoing concerns with a rare tumor disorder (Carney triad), and osteoporosis. I learned to see myself as graceful and elegant, at ease with dancing, and with sparkling shoes and dazzling outfits.

Learning to dance made me bolder about taking new risks and influenced my creative rhythms, leading the way to writing. When an adult education class on writing caught my eye, I enrolled. Always a writer of letters, journals, newsletter articles, and professional reports, I longed to craft creative pieces and expand my options for inspiring others. Similarities between dancing and writing soon emerged: developing patterns, trying variations, capturing the theme and mood, following the lead of an idea. Words dance. Sometimes they waltz, sometimes they swing and sway, and sometimes they speak with a staccato tempo.

When offered early retirement four years ago, I took it and didn't look back. The decision felt right, an opportunity to join Bill in retirement and to pursue more writing dreams—daring to share my work and offer it for publication.

Following my husband's lead to try dancing all those years ago has resulted in major gains for our health and happiness.

We continued dancing because it put a positive spin on our lives and kept us active and motivated, big benefits to transfer from work to retired lives. How grateful I am for Bill's whole-hearted support for both my dancing and writing. I would have missed out big time had I not pursued what first seemed unreachable.

I continue to grow and try out new possibilities. Dancing keeps my life on beat and my brain and body going strong. It took patience, practice, and persistence, but now dancing, along with writing, ranks as one of my greatest accomplishments and sources of joy. Sometimes the hardest tasks allow us to become our best.

— Ronda Armstrong —

Hope for the Best
and *Expect* the Best

Introduction

Happy people like candy bars. At least according to most Snickers commercials and a 2011 *Journal of Consumer Research* article, which found that people who report being "happy" are more apt to eat candy bars. "Hopeful" people, on the other hand, were more inclined to choose a healthier option, like an apple. Why? Hope focuses on future-oriented thinking, while the characteristic focus of happiness is on past positive experiences. So if you want to learn to eat healthier in the future and for the future, deliberately focus more on good things in life that are to come and a little less on your wonderful past.

The growing area of positive psychology purports that optimism plays a vital role in helping promote healthy behaviors. Researchers have concluded that optimists make future-oriented choices that encourage good health, like the aforementioned eating of fruit. They have a knack for making healthy decisions in the present that will positively affect the future. Exercising today, knowing it will pay off down the road, is another excellent example. Even in the face of a health crisis, many optimists tend to cope and adjust to new circumstances better than their not-so-optimistic counterparts. Further, a

2011 meta-analytic study undertaken by researchers at Denison University examined 52 different research articles focusing on resilience, finding that hope and optimism were key factors in helping people maintain or reestablish their psychological well-being when facing difficult life circumstances such as physical illness.

Unlike clinical psychology, which looks at pathology and problems, positive psychology emphasizes constructive thoughts and actions. I wholeheartedly agree with the last positive sentence of Ronda Armstrong's dancing and writing story, which reads: "Sometimes the hardest tasks allow us to become our best." Maintaining positivity, however, can be a difficult task when it comes to health problems. In the face of medical difficulties that can seem insurmountable, some people are quick to give up on encouraging sayings like "Good things come to those who wait" or "Patience is a virtue." And sometimes we simply don't win the health battle. Research is clear about the role that hope and optimism play in healthy lifestyles and recovery from illness.

Throughout my years in practice, I've met with countless individuals who have given up on their health. They've abandoned hope of ever having a baby, decided the extra weight will never come off, or let the helplessness created by painful fibromyalgia win out in the long run. You and I both know health challenges can be particularly complex, and once you give up, it can be even more difficult to recover. I've also seen patients develop a healthy mindset in the face of health adversity. With that in mind, you'll find a few recommendations in this chapter for you to employ as you strive to protect the hope and optimism necessary for great health.

Keep Your Identity

Perhaps the largest single loss anyone can face when dealing with poor health is the loss of individual identity. No one wants to trade who they are for a list of diagnoses, blood work, test results, or a prognosis. It seems so inhuman to rearrange our lives for a set of symptoms. If you are struggling with a health-related condition, don't let that illness become the factor that describes you better than anything else.

Decide now that you are a person and not a medical condition. Just like I tell my patients, if you have a cough, runny nose, and sneeze a lot, you do not become a cold. You are simply a person with a cold. If it seems health concerns are rocking your identity boat, then it's important to grieve that loss so you can regain your sense of self. In another Chicken Soup for the Soul book I wrote called *Chicken Soup for the Soul: Say Goodbye to Stress*, I dedicated an entire chapter to loss, grief, and the stress they both create. In order to wade through the loss of identity, you should confide in a spouse, close friend, or therapist. Your brain is wired so that grieving is natural and restorative. But when we prevent grieving from happening, we exacerbate stress and likely deepen the identity problem at hand.

One of the ways you can unknowingly give up your identity is to talk constantly about the wearisome issues facing you. Now before you correct me and question whether I am a kindhearted psychologist, I agree wholeheartedly that it's important to talk about the emotions, thoughts, and behaviors related to any medical issue that you're confronting. I am just encouraging you to keep your identity and let the people around you continue to experience you as a real person rather than a diagnosis. It is very meaningful when you have friends who care about your health. You should be thankful to them for their concern. Don't forget to joke with them at the coffee shop, swap ideas about the latest romance novel, sing in the community chorus, head up the volunteer program at your church or temple, or get lost in a dazzling jazz mix on a rainy afternoon. If you lose yourself, you will lose hope and optimism—and others will miss you, too.

Prepare Exclusively for Success

Regardless of the odds facing you and your health, setting yourself up for success can lead to positive, confident feelings. How you think about your own health and health management is critical. This is where the alliance you've forged with your brain should stand front and center. My favorite example about creating a mindset that sets up success doesn't come from one of my patients, but from a dear friend and former neighbor who my wife and I adore.

One late afternoon, the telephone rang. Our good friend Andy (that's the moniker Anne has had ever since my son Grant misspoke her name when he was learning to talk) called to tell us she had been through a series of tests after experiencing some unpleasant symptoms. She had been diagnosed with colorectal cancer and would be starting treatment within the week at Massachusetts General Hospital in Boston. It was difficult to digest this news given its unexpected nature. But also unforeseen was the unique twist Andy assigned to her dilemma and treatment protocol.

After wading through some healthy denial, which allowed her some time to sort through options and absorb the shock of her diagnosis, she created a mindset for her future. She told us she had instructed her treatment team to avoid sharing statistics or probabilities with her. She agreed that while some people would want to know that information, she believed it would be useless for her plan of attack. Andy's attitude was positive and she was planning to do everything possible to beat the cancer. Knowing treatment success rates, and by default rates about failure, would only interfere with her healthy mindset by leading to anxiety, depression, and helplessness. She wanted to keep her head serene and upbeat. Notice the tone of optimism in Andy's plan?

Really, her cognitive plan made good sense. For her, any time that would have been given to negative thoughts would now be spent staying positive and planning for the future of her treatment. If you're trying to create a positive outlook, you might want to follow Andy's lead and check the bad news at the door. Whether your health circumstance is dire or a mere matter of maintenance, doing all you can to promote your health can be reassuring and may offer the confidence boost you need when things get tough. Like Andy said, "I am going to fight this cancer regardless of whether statistics indicate things are good or bad. For me the fight will be the same." And fight, she did. After several months of chemotherapy and radiation, losing some hair and weight, and maintaining hope and optimism through friendships and prayer, Andy was cancer free.

Build the Right Kind of Support

The types of support people need throughout life vary. In 1954, personality theorist Abraham Maslow described how self-actualized individuals, those individuals who have fully met their psychological and physical needs, only need a handful of close friends. Since that time, other researchers have striven to make Maslow's ideas contemporary, but the fact remains: humans have basic needs. If you notice the personality model mapped out on an image of Maslow's pyramid on the next page, you'll see one level that focuses on love and belonging. Humans need to connect to others and belong to groups. Many learn connecting skills as children, and then use them throughout adolescence and into adulthood.

Consider the variety of organizations and clubs you can belong to: social clubs, volunteer organizations, churches, book clubs, hobby groups, sports teams. And the list goes on. Having social connections in myriad ways and connecting with others who have similar health concerns can create a unique bond between individuals. Allowing new people into your life can be beneficial as well. Think of your social network being structured like an athletic team aimed for a championship playoff game.

Each member has different skills, all of you have the same goal, and encouragement is offered freely. Choose teammates who can pick you up and keep the game going even when you want a timeout or hit a wall. A cohesive team keeps its eyes on the ultimate goal and is willing to go into overtime or extra innings to help you protect hope.

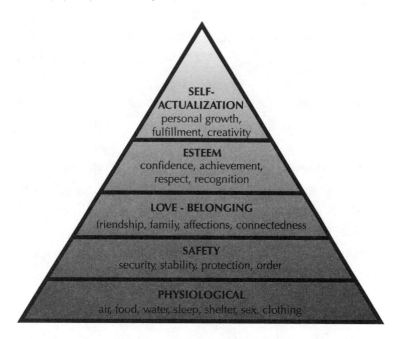

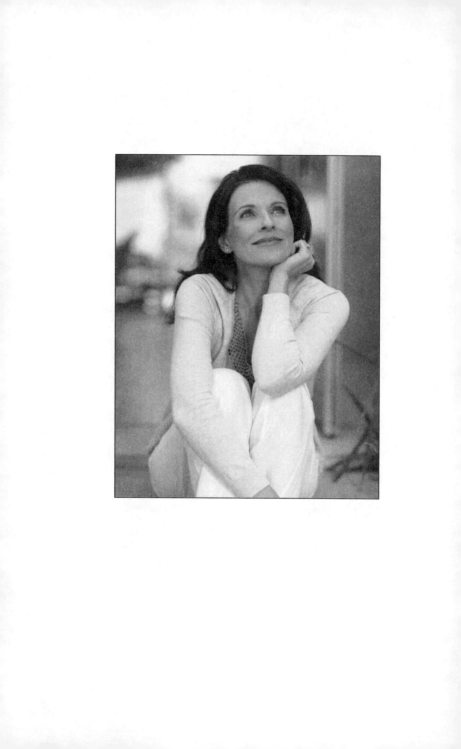

Chapter 4
Dr. Seuss, Kevorkian or Oz: Connecting with the Right Doctor

It Takes Two
to Tango

Hearing Bonnie describe her situation, I understood her embarrassment. Television shows, movies and books rarely portray characters using the bathroom. If they do, it is often in some exaggerated, offensive, or comical way. There is a general avoidance of acknowledging human bodily functions. But we all pee. There was some irony here for Bonnie, a writer and producer for the television industry.

Bonnie had a performance-based anxiety called paruresis, or "shy bladder." Affecting seven percent of the country, paruresis is the fear of urinating in public restrooms. She faced symptoms of worry, embarrassment, dread and humiliation. Bonnie felt severe anxiety, and usually could not go at all, when faced with having to pee anywhere but the privacy of her own home. She worried what others would think about her if they saw her go into a bathroom, or, far worse, heard her doing her business in there.

By the time she graduated from college, Bonnie's shy bladder had taken over her life. "What took you so long in there?" A joking comment from her first boss psychologically nagged at Bonnie for years. To avoid wondering what her colleagues would think, she avoided leaving a long meeting or a table at lunch to use the bathroom, even when she really had to go. If she ever found herself in a restroom at the same time as another person, Bonnie felt preoccupied with worry about what the person might be thinking about her, the sounds she was making, and even the duration of her urine stream. She would even splash the water in the toilet so it would sound like she was peeing to anyone else who might hear her. She knew this was excessive and unreasonable, and felt angry with herself for worrying about something others barely think about.

She was afraid to tell her colleagues, family, friends, and even her primary care doctor about her embarrassing problem. She thought she would be seen as weak. She felt like a fraud, burdened by her secret. She turned down social and recreational activities she loved, to avoid public restrooms. Bonnie lived her restricted life for years before finally coming to my office one February morning to begin cognitive behavioral therapy.

Bonnie struggled to tell me her story, covering her face and squirming in her seat. "I've never talked about this with anyone," she told me. There was a long pause as she collected her thoughts. I assured her that she could take her time. Finally, she began, "I want to dance at my daughter's wedding. I can't let her down." Her daughter, Maggie, was planning a destination wedding in Tahiti. "But I can't go, because I can't... I can't... pee in public," she finally blurted out. Then, "Oh! I meant I can't use public restrooms." Her face flushed scarlet. Then, to my surprise, she giggled. I smiled and assured her I knew what she meant, and that I had helped others with paruresis. She looked relieved.

With encouragement, Bonnie was able to tell me more details of what she had been experiencing all these years: when it started, the many things she had come to avoid, how she learned to hide her problem, and how sad and afraid it made her feel inside. She told me about the "crazy thoughts" that plagued her. Bonnie was in tears as the pain and shame she had been shouldering poured out. She expressed relief after sharing her anguish. "I just want to be like everyone else, not a bathroom obsessed lunatic." She could not fathom the idea of the long plane ride to Tahiti, and all the public restrooms along the way. The wedding was in July, less than six months away.

She was ready to tackle her shy bladder with professional help. She agreed to keep a thought journal to capture thoughts like "I'm less of a person because of my bladder issue" and "what if my bladder bursts and the pilot has to make an emergency landing?" She made the commitment to document all these ideas, no matter how difficult. I encouraged her to be as detailed as possible, so that we could work with even the most embarrassing thoughts. Each week, we reviewed the journal, and together, examined the accuracy, logic and likelihood of each thought in order to challenge her assumptions.

Bonnie found it easier and easier to share what was on her mind. She began to think about herself much more positively. She referred to me as her partner in a dance she called the "tinkle tango," helping her get ready for the bigger dance that was fast approaching. She also agreed to "experiments" that allowed her to test out new coping skills and practice being in and around bathrooms in restaurants, grocery stores and then the mall. She even made a trip to the airport just to use the restroom. I genuinely admired her openness and determination, and the trust she placed in me. She exceeded both our expectations, and we were hopeful when she left for her trip. Bonnie knew she could count on me as her partner.

Near the end of that summer, I received a manila envelope postmarked from overseas. Inside was a photo of Bonnie, in a conga line, beaming as she stood behind a beautiful bride. "Dear Dr. Brown," said the enclosed note, "as you can see, I am way beyond the tinkle tango! Our work together has reopened a world of possibilities for me. Many thanks, Bonnie."

— Felicia F. Brown, Ph.D. —

The Break

I was thirty-four that night in May 1978 when my sons and I jumped from my second floor bedroom window to our dark back yard below. We were escaping two men who battered down the door to our San Francisco apartment, in what the police later said was probably a drug-induced rage.

Brad, my fifteen-year-old, dropped to the ground easily, and helped his eleven-year-old brother Doug up from where he landed on the grass. I hesitated, terrified of heights. But when the pounding on the door intensified, I followed, stiff-legged with fear—landing on my feet on the concrete back step—crying out as a searing pain shot through my left ankle. I heard the wail of police sirens coming close to our house. Someone called the police, I thought, as I collapsed on the ground. The paramedics loaded us into an ambulance and rushed to St. Francis Memorial Hospital.

"You're going to be all right, Mom, I know it," Brad said, taking my hand.

"Promise, Mom?" Doug pleaded, his face pale.

I'd asked the police to call my best friend Kerry; she arrived at the hospital soon after we did. "What a nightmare," she said, hugging me, "but somehow we'll get through it. Don't worry about the boys; they'll come home with me. Get some rest."

The orthopedic surgeon studied the X-rays of my foot and ankle carefully before speaking. "I won't lie to you. You have a serious injury, with bones crunched together from impact, here and here," he said, indicating where on the X-ray, "and severe dislocation, here and here. I think closed reduction, without surgery, is your best option—less chance of infection, no pins, and no scars."

He shook his head, looking solemn. "I'll do what I can, but you should be prepared that, at best, you'll probably walk with a significant limp."

The doctor's pessimistic tone was chilling. I could barely take it all in—my home broken into, my family threatened, and now maybe a permanently damaged ankle.

I'm a single mom, I thought; I support a family. What will become of us if I can't work? And why did this happen to me? I'm a glass-half-full person by nature. Since moving to San Francisco after my divorce two years earlier, I had taken classes on the power of positive thinking, and visualization—and living life, unafraid.

The fear lessened as these thoughts went through my mind. I took a long deep breath and as I released it—from somewhere deep inside me, something flared, hot and bright with determination.

And a clear, calm voice within me said "NO!"

"Don't worry doctor," I heard myself say. "With your skill and my will, I'll be fine."

The closed reduction was done the next morning. When I woke from the anesthesia, Kerry and my sons were waiting. My left leg—which burned like it was on fire—was encased in a plaster cast to my groin. Eight days later I went home in a wheelchair.

I spent six weeks in the huge, cumbersome cast. It was so immobilizing I used a walker to drag it, painfully, around my house. Couldn't walk, couldn't drive, couldn't go out and earn my living—I'd never felt so helpless in my life.

I filled out police reports but the men who broke in weren't found. Police surveillance in our immediate neighborhood increased, which I appreciated. But my gut feeling (which turned out to be right) was I'd suffered a random misfortune, and the intruders wouldn't return.

Luckily for my family, Kerry moved in to take care of us for six weeks until the full cast came off. It was replaced, for two more months, by a lighter, knee-high one—which enabled me to hobble around on crutches and drive my car again—and although still in pain, I'd gained enough strength to return to work. The boys and I had some sessions with a therapist to talk through our feelings about the break-in and its impact on our lives.

And I focused, every day, on remaining unafraid.

The doctor, still noncommittal, stared at the X-rays three and a half months after my injury.

"We'll see," was all he'd promise.

Despite my best intentions I was horrified by my weak, withered left leg, which hurt terribly and buckled under me when I took my first steps after the cast came off. A few days later I began strengthening my leg muscles by walking barefoot in the sand at Ocean Beach. Brad and Doug went with me after school, and as I struggled to put one foot in front of the other—a son supporting me on either side—I visualized myself in my favorite platform heels with a knee-length skirt swinging gracefully around my legs.

I saw myself dancing.

One year after my injury I waltzed into the doctor's office for my final checkup wearing platform heels and a knee-length skirt. Aside from some minor nerve damage causing a pins-and-needles sensation on top of my foot, the physical aftereffects of my jump from the window were a slightly thickened left ankle and a foot that couldn't point enough to stand on my toes.

I'd never be a ballerina—but I'd dance.

The doctor's face registered amazement. He shook his head. "No limp," he said, watching me walk. "Remarkable."

I smiled and nodded. We were partners, I thought gratefully. We each did our job well.

"I told you, doctor—with your skill and my will, I'll be fine."

~ Lynn Sunday ~

A Healing
Bedside Manner

"I'm sorry, what did you say?"

The doctor stood before me, a tall man, but short on personality and sporting a solemn expression. "You have systemic lupus," he said matter-of-factly.

I must have looked at him like he was speaking a foreign language.

"Lupus," he reiterated, "is an autoimmune disease. The antibodies that exist in your body to fight off disease actually get confused and attack your healthy cells." He went on to try to explain all the complications associated with the disease. I remember certain details but mostly I remember him telling me not to have any more children as childbirth would jumpstart additional symptoms. Symptoms that could be potentially life threatening.

As I got up to leave, shaken and thoroughly drained, he said his parting words, "And I would discourage any further research. There is no cure and there is nothing you can do to prevent its progression."

Needless to say, I did research lupus and its symptoms—fatigue, joint pain and swelling—were all consistent with what I was experiencing. The prognosis: chronic pain, and eventually some major organs could be affected, which could cause shutdown and possible death. Definitely not words that a thirty-three-year-old mother of two wants to hear.

I sought homeopathic remedies online. I found out that echinacea had a proven track record in strengthening one's immune system. I decided that along with the herb I would strengthen my mindset by immersing myself in my family. My son was less than a year old and my daughter was three. It was an incredibly active time, especially for someone feeling anything but active.

After one follow-up visit with the same doctor, I felt lost and alone and decided never to go back to him. The years passed. When I would feel tired and achy I did my best to find time to rest. I pulled strength from my children and their laughter.

Finally, after many years, I went to an internist who had been recommended by a friend.

The first time I met Dr. K I was instantly drawn to her. She was petite, with warm brown eyes and a firm handshake.

"Anna, so nice to meet you."

I remember her standing there holding my hand and looking into my eyes, not at a clipboard. She was looking at me.

"So, let's talk a little."

Instantly my defenses were down. Before I knew it, she had me running on and on about my children, my husband, my life and dreams. I told her about all the activities I was involved in.

"I'm tired just hearing about all you do," Dr. K said with a laugh.

She looked at the papers I had filled out and said, "Lupus? When were you diagnosed with lupus?"

"About eight years ago, when my son was an infant."

She looked a little confused. "Judging by what you are telling me I would say it is highly unlikely that you have lupus. We'll run some tests and see what's going on."

"If I don't have lupus, what do I have?" I asked. Had I been making up the symptoms all this time?

"I don't have that answer right now, but you can be sure we won't stop until we find out. You and me together."

After several rounds of tests, more targeted questions and greater research into my family history, we came to some conclusive answers. One being that I did not have systemic lupus.

I didn't know whether I should jump for joy or scream because I had been living the last eight years in fear of a potentially fatal disease. I felt foolish for believing in a doctor who had made me feel so uncomfortable. One who had discouraged conversation.

But then I realized that I had been living every day, not so much in fear, but happiness. Every day was a gift and I knew it.

Dr. K has taught me the importance of open communication for continued good health. Previously, it was difficult to talk about my ailments and pinpoint my concerns. Now when I go to see her, or any specialist, I prepare a list of problems and questions so I don't forget anything. I've even taken to putting a small x where the pain is so I can immediately point to the problem area.

I love Dr. K. I love her demeanor, and in a world of overworked, mechanical doctors, she emanates a wonderful bedside manner that encourages healing. I trust her with my health and the health of my family. And I consider her a great friend.

~ Anna Koopman ~

Dr. Seuss, Kevorkian or Oz: Connecting with the Right Doctor

Introduction

Many people believe psychologists choose their profession because they enjoy helping people. For me, helping people is actually a wonderful byproduct of what I truly love most about being a psychologist, and that is problem solving. I'm reminded of another groaner psychologist joke about problem solving. The patient said to his psychologist, "Doctor, I think I might be a wheelbarrow." "Well," the therapist instructed, "don't let people push you around!" In reality, problem solving isn't *that* easy and requires much more collaboration than a one-sentence punch line. By the way, "good" humor in therapy is completely acceptable!

Both doctor and patient should aspire to a collaboration that is just as cohesive as the connection between mind and body. Just like the lyrics of the song, "love and marriage go together like a horse and carriage," your physical and psychological structures should go hand in hand, too. And it's up to you to get them to communicate with each other. The significant, collaborative relationship you have with your doctor can have a lot to do with your satisfaction and positive healthcare outcomes, too.

Building a good relationship with your primary healthcare provider can happen and should be something most individuals aspire to. Research reveals how a strong doctor-patient relationship can affect your health positively. For example, in a 2010 article published in the *Journal of General Internal Medicine*, Professor Alan Christensen suggests that when doctors and their patients have similar attitudes about treatment and conditions, patients are more likely to keep their prescriptions refilled. Such a phenomenon increases treatment adherence for patients and, I'm sure, keeps doctors pleased at the same time.

Get on the Same Page

Fortunately, the number of studies about the psychology of relationships and the potential benefits that can be gained by an individual seeking treatment are growing. Decades of social psychological research have amply established that the more similar you are to people, the more apt you are to be drawn to them. Of course, this does not mean that if there are vast differences between you and your physician, the relationship is doomed. Some of the richest therapeutic relationships I have had with patients included differences between us that were quite distinct, even obvious. But, in spite of those differences, those relationships were allowed to flourish because we shared and appreciated the value of obvious difference—something we shared and a value we had in common.

Simply put, the more you have in common with your provider, the more likely you will adhere to treatment recommendations and instructions. Once you are headed in the direction of having an exceptional fit with your healthcare provider, you should begin to prioritize effective communication skills so you can be on your way to promoting healthier outcomes. You might ask yourself, how would I ever develop a good relationship with my physician, especially when our face-to-face time is already so brief? A strong alliance can be built with some intentional planning and strategy.

Build an Alliance with Your Doctor Through Communication

1. Get to know your doctor as soon as you can.

Unfortunately, too many people meet their physician for the first time when they are in crisis. To help open up good communication, set up a nonmedical appointment with your new physician just to get to know one another before a crisis hits. While you may feel a bit silly going to the doctor without having an actual medical problem, most physicians will appreciate that you're taking time to get to know them. During that first informational meeting be sure to specifically talk about communication and how your physician prefers to hear from you. At the same time, don't hesitate to let him or her know how you like to receive information as well.

2. E-mail your doctor to open up lines of communication.

In 2010, Kaiser Permanente looked at over 35,000 of their patients and discovered those diagnosed with diabetes, hypertension, or some combination of both had a better healthcare outcome when they communicated with their doctors via secure e-mail. Obviously positive outcomes in this study had little to do with technology, and everything to do with the fact that patients had increased communication with their physicians because of e-mail. Opening up lines of communication is critical. It is likely that through e-mail, doctor-patient communication was stronger.

You impact your health positively by opening up different avenues of communication with your physician. If she does indeed welcome e-mails, find out her e-mail address and whether she uses it regularly. Perhaps the hospital, clinic, or other healthcare system your doctor works in has a communication portal just for this purpose. Find out if your doctor is someone who is available around the clock or if she has someone who pinch-hits for her over the weekends. Different healthcare organizations have different policies addressing e-mail communication, so be sure you understand what the organization's expectations are. Also, try to meet staff and other liaisons who are links between your doctor and you.

3. Have realistic expectations for communication.

As a psychologist, I've had the opportunity to work with many physicians, play a role in their training, and know them socially. I've paid attention to what physicians are like from those experiences, but truth be told, I've learned the most from the physicians who have been my clinical patients. I've heard about the stress at home, the long work hours, the demands of insurance companies, the frustration of career challenges, and the list goes on. As we discuss the benefits of good interactions, it's important to keep in mind that your physician is a human being just like you. Just like the demands of your job, the demands of healthcare are greater than ever, too. Both of you are under pressure, just different kinds of pressure.

If you know you are the type of person who needs immediate feedback, explicit directions or has frequent medical concerns, choose a physician who is a similar type of communicator. If not, I can guarantee your expectations about communication will go unmet. Don't put yourself in that situation. It's okay for you to continue to search for a physician who matches your communication style well. Just remember, however, that no one, including your physician, is a perfect communicator. Healthcare is a blend of science and personality. Whether you prioritize bedside manner, medical school training, or faith beliefs, keep searching for the individual with whom you can communicate well.

4. Be prepared for your office visits.

I communicate better with my wife when I think about what I'm trying to tell her before I say anything. Just ask her! Admittedly, I can blurt things out from time to time, which only clouds the message I'm actually trying to convey. The same goes for you and your physician. When you know you're getting ready to have a conversation, spend some time preparing your message. Make it clear, thorough, and concise. In fact, it is just fine for you to write down the points you'd like to make so you don't forget them during your appointment. Just don't create an overwhelming document that's so exhaustive it is useless to both of you. Feel free to hand your doctor a copy of the notes you've prepared prior to your appointment so he'll have a record of your concerns and questions. I always appreciate a patient who arrives for therapy with notes in hand and a reading copy for me. It literally keeps us on the same page.

5. Be honest about everything.

When it comes to communication, this is the toughest part. Honesty. When developing any healthy, useful relationship with a healthcare provider, honesty is necessary. Remember Bonnie? She valiantly (and eventually) confided in Felicia Brown about her paralyzing embarrassment when using public restroom facilities. She relied on the confidential relationship she had with Felicia so she could make strides to trump her disorder. For Bonnie and for you, doctor-patient confidentiality is a legal concept created for your benefit and provides plenty of room to speak freely. While the limits of confidentiality can vary from state to state, the spirit of confidentiality remains the same. I have spoken with hundreds of individuals in my practice about very sensitive topics and agree it can be difficult to talk about personal or intimate topics such as sexually transmitted diseases, sexual dysfunction, certain types of habits, or specific medical concerns.

Dealing with body parts which are rarely discussed with others, let alone with a stranger, can be challenging. It is not just the physical unmentionables that can be tough to be honest about. Sometimes patients have difficulty sharing information they believe will change the physician's perspective about them. For example, a patient may misuse prescription medication or under-report behaviors such as alcohol or marijuana use, recreational sex, or an eating disorder. Honesty has been the best policy for a long time, and it certainly applies to your healthcare. Remember, the goal is to improve your health.

As a springboard to more open and honest communication, you can start off a conversation about a sensitive topic by saying, "I guess I am going to have to take a risk and tell you about…" Once you start to understand that your physician has literally heard it all, you'll feel calmer about being honest, and your dialogue will be enhanced. In Chapter 8, you'll read about even more ways of taking charge of embarrassment and using it to your healthcare advantage.

6. Speak assertively and directly about what you believe.

In 2010, researchers at Texas A&M University and the

Pennsylvania State University College of Medicine provided some insightful information about how some doctors perceive their patients' understanding of their healthcare. The research suggests physicians in general are probably not highly skilled at assessing what their patients believe about healthcare. What does this mean for you? It means you should speak up and discuss your beliefs with your doctor. By doing so, you're informing him or her more about the backdrop of your life, which can include values, faith, family history, and even misconceptions about types of treatments. When you deliberately offer this information to your physician, she will be better positioned to give you customized treatment and educate you about what she believes your healthiest goals should be.

Art Appreciation: 101

Did you know medical schools such as Harvard, Yale and Cornell now offer their students art appreciation courses? It's believed that observation and the critical examination of art will strengthen a doctor's ability to pay attention to small details in patients, ultimately enhancing case conceptualization, system understanding and patient care.

If You Can, Choose a Healthy Doctor

Remember the slogan that used to be printed on milk cartons in the school cafeteria, "You are what you eat." That phrase stands true today and certainly applies to your physician. Research conducted at the University of Michigan suggests doctors' own health behaviors, including eating right and exercising often, affect how they counsel patients on the same topics. It appears that doctors who are living healthy lifestyles are more apt to be confident when counseling patients about the same. And it stands to reason the message physicians are sending is far more believable when they are also living proof. In today's collaborative medical culture, it is appropriate to ask your doctors about their own health habits. However, don't expect them to discuss highly sensitive or intimate information with you.

Many of my patients have similar health regimens as I have. They may share the latest healthy snack recipe they've found, while I may suggest to them a new route for running or biking that I have discovered. It's also fun to share ideas about smartphone apps that target healthy thinking and living. Once you're convinced you're on the same health wavelength, you will probably find it helpful to share your health habits with your physician. Discovering such similarities may strengthen your alliance, ultimately affecting your personal health in a positive way.

It's Okay to Say Goodbye to Your Physician

Even with good effort on both of your parts, sometimes a doctor-patient relationship just doesn't work out. Making a decision to change doctors or healthcare providers, particularly when you are in the midst of an immediate healthcare concern, can be difficult. Sometimes patients want to move on to another professional but don't know how to broach the topic with their current doctor. It's not uncommon to fear that you'll offend your physician or appear as though you don't appreciate all that's already been done for you. But how do you know it's time to look for a new doctor? The following are a few red flags that indicate the relationship needs to be evaluated seriously.

1. Your provider seems frustrated with you.
2. The relationship chemistry you once had changes dramatically.
3. Your physician is offended if you ask for a second opinion.
4. You routinely disagree with your physician's recommendations.
5. Your physician does not value your input when making treatment decisions.
6. You notice feelings of resentment toward your provider.
7. Your compliance with treatment recommendations decreases or is nonexistent.

If you make the decision that you must move on to a new provider, be sure to have closure with your current physician. You may want to acknowledge the efforts displayed on your behalf with a written note or some sort of verbal recognition at your last appointment. Then, do your research to find another doctor. Sometimes the provider you are saying goodbye to can make referrals to colleagues on your behalf, particularly if the individual you have been seeing is a specialist. Don't hesitate to get referrals from friends and family, too. Since your friends are probably a lot like you, the fit they have with their doctor may very well be a good fit for you too.

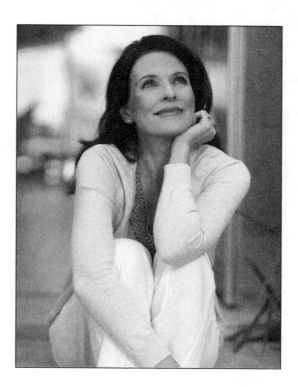

Chapter 5
Brain Strategies for Robust Living

A Positive Road
to Recovery

I never thought about what my mind could do for me when it came to my body being ill. My usual reaction to an illness or an injury was to try not to think about it, to put it to the back of my mind and try not to focus on such things as pain, misery, or inability. This kind of reaction helped me through a lot of minor ailments, but failed me completely when it came to facing the heart problems that eventually overtook me. Coping with that situation required a more positive approach to healing.

I thought I was in perfect health when I suffered the aortic dissection. I was on the verge of death when I arrived at the hospital, and after the doctors assessed that I was too weak for an arterial transplant they put me in a deep coma for two weeks and hoped my body would stabilize itself. When I finally woke up in intensive care it was to the news that my life had changed forever.

Back home I was unable to get out of bed. The pain was intense and every time I tried to move the stress would shoot my blood pressure up to dangerous levels. The massive amounts of medication I required to keep my heart rate and pressure subdued and my blood pressure under control made it almost impossible to think straight or concentrate on anything.

Whenever I closed my eyes I was assailed by nightmarish visions that were a side effect of the drugs. My prognosis wasn't good, my odds were short at surviving my condition, and my options were almost nonexistent. Life began to be a losing battle.

Then one night as I lay in bed, I realized this illness of mine was something I could not run away from. This was a disease that would kill me if I let it control my life. I had to find a way to deal with all the pain and misery I was going through. I prayed to God for the strength to deal with this new burden. It came to me that I was not a quitter. Whenever life had given me a challenge I'd found a positive way to deal with it. So that was what I would do with my illness.

Instead of just lying there telling myself there was nothing I could do, I decided to take action. The next morning I made myself sit on the edge of the bed. I looked out the bedroom window and watched as the clouds rolled past in a bright blue sky. I told myself, "In a week I'm going to go outside and breathe that fresh air for myself."

The next few days I spent my time talking with my family, letting them know that I wanted them to feel free to visit any time they wanted, encouraging them to treat me as someone on the road to recovery. I began to focus on everything around me, telling myself the fog and confusion caused by my medication was something I could handle. Slowly, a bit at a time, I was able to concentrate again.

I made a game of setting a new goal for myself each day. By the third day I stood outside and drew in a breath of fresh air. I told myself I wasn't going to dread each visit to the doctor or every scan or X-ray the specialists took. I told myself the results would be positive. I followed the limitations the doctors placed on me for a while, but slowly, as I eased myself back into my life, I found those limitations stretched, and the strength and health to handle them.

I don't want to give the impression there weren't any setbacks. Many times I found my heart suddenly beating wildly and dizziness forcing me to my knees. At first this kind of reaction meant a sudden trip to the hospital, but gradually, I told myself that I could handle such episodes, and as they came on I told myself that I would be calm, that this was a natural part of the disease and I wasn't in any real danger, that I could control the reactions my body was having.

My mind and my body began to work together to help me cope with this disease. I developed routines where I would calm myself, will my heartbeat to return to normal and try to even things out. I found that I could slowly and safely increase my physical activity and that I could take on many of the responsibilities I'd had before the attack. I was careful to always take my medication, get enough rest, and not push things too far, but this was something more. This was my mind taking positive steps to help control and guide my recovery. It worked wonders.

Over a decade has passed since my life was changed by my illness, and I'm happy to say that I've regained much of what I'd lost before. There are changes, things I still have to deal with, but now I deal with them directly and positively, with the knowledge that there is much I can do to help myself by how I think about myself, and how I handle each situation as it arises. I'm on a much more positive path in my life, and having that attitude has made the journey that much more enjoyable.

— John P. Buentello —

The White Light

"**Y**ou're next," announced the radiation technician. "Just walk straight down the hall until you reach the double doors and turn right."

"Can my husband go with me?" I asked, hesitantly.

"No, I'm sorry—patients only!"

My husband of twenty years, Mark, blew me a kiss and watched as I caught it in mid-air, clutching it close to my heart. It was our signal to each other that everything was going to be okay.

Radiation was the last of a three-part series in the treatment for breast cancer, but it was what I feared the most. It was the reason why I didn't get a mammogram at age forty; I was terrified of its "harmful" effects.

The long corridor leading to the treatment room had "DANGER" signs posted along its sterile walls, which further fueled my fears. The technician who followed closely behind me had a kind smile and a soothing voice, but nothing could calm the terror that I felt.

Once inside the treatment area, the thick concrete walls closed in on me. My heart raced and beads of sweat formed on my upper lip as the nurse tried to make me comfortable. "Don't worry," she said. "Everyone feels this way the first time; you'll be just fine."

I didn't believe her!

After the technician placed me on the exam table, she warned me not to move. "Here's the panic button, just in case you need it," she said with a warm smile. "We'll continue to communicate through the intercom system and treatment will start when you see the red light flash."

Too paralyzed to speak, I nodded my head "yes" to her request. As soon as she left my side, my body went into spasm. How was I going to lie still for ten minutes? What if I accidentally moved and the radiation targeted my eye. Would I go blind? What if I sneezed or had to cough?

As soon as the red light flashed to signal "radiation in progress" my body froze and a tear tickled down my cheek. "Don't move!" shouted the technician. "We're almost done," she reassured.

Five minutes later the technician popped back in and announced, "See, that wasn't so bad, was it?" My tear stained cheeks went unnoticed as she helped me up from the exam table. "I'll see you tomorrow at the same time," she said.

The technician led me back to the dressing room area where I changed out of my blue-and-white checkered gown with the "sexy" back slit and placed it in the tub marked "red" for radiation. As I contemplated my fate for the next six weeks, I couldn't help but notice the lovely woman sitting in the waiting room with a cheerful smile. She was sporting a bright pink terrycloth bandana—a symbol that she too was a patient.

She smiled warmly and said, "I guess we'll be seeing a lot of each other for the next few weeks—right?"

I wanted to run out the door, but I stopped and replied, "Yes, I think we're going to be bosom buddies."

She giggled and smiled. "Hi, I'm Patty and I'm a regular around here! They've given me six months to live, but I'm trying to make every moment count. I have six children at home who need me, so I'm sticking around," she announced without blinking.

The lump in my throat didn't permit me to speak. I nodded my head while forcing back the tears. And then—as if someone had patted me on the back to let the lump pass—I asked, "How do you remain so positive?"

There was a long pause, followed by the words, "I have a little mantra that I use when I'm going through radiation and it works for me." Patty shared how she repeated the words: "This white light is curing my cancer. I imagine that the light is piercing each one of the cancer cells and is destroying them." Patty grabbed my hand tightly and announced, "Welcome to the sorority none of us wanted to join!"

I stood motionless as she explained her methodology and then I asked, "Do you mind if I borrow your mantra?"

Patty laughed and said, "Of course you can; it's simple and you'll find that the time will pass quickly. See you tomorrow," she offered, cheerfully.

I thought about what Patty said and waited until I got out into the parking lot to practice my new "cure" for cancer.

Positive thinking with positive imagery, that's how I would get through the next thirty-six treatments.

While driving home, I practiced, "This white light is curing my cancer!"

The following day, I was only half as fearful as the day before. As the technician positioned my body on the exam table, I repeated the words softly, "This white light is curing my cancer."

"Remember, you need to lie perfectly still," the technician admonished.

I blinked "yes" and continued with shallow breathing and repeated the words, "This white light is curing my cancer."

After my second treatment, I felt even more confident. I couldn't wait to share the good news with Patty. She was easy to spot in the waiting room with her bright pink turban.

"How did it go?" Patty asked.

"Perfectly, I think I'm cured!" I responded.

Patty chuckled and replied, "Now you've got the idea!"

The next six weeks passed quickly as I got into a routine and synchronized my thoughts with treatment. The fear of radiation was gone and instead I looked forward to the "white" light that was curing my cancer.

On my last day of treatment, the radiation oncologist shared with me that I didn't need to see him again—unless I wanted to. I assured him that I had no plans of returning! He shook my hand and led me out into the waiting room where there was a team of nurses and technicians holding a bouquet of white balloons. Too overwhelmed to speak, I allowed the tears to trickle down my cheeks. One of the nurses slid a white balloon into my hand and led me into the parking lot. My "bosom buddy" Patty was by my side. On the count of three, we released the balloons and watched as they became points of light against the clear blue sky.

It's been fifteen years since I stood in the hospital parking lot and released a single white balloon, but I've never let go of the lessons that cancer has taught me. Every year when I return for my annual mammogram, a remnant of fear tries to wiggle back in. And when that happens, I know exactly what to do. I take a deep breath and whisper the words, "This white light has cured my cancer!"

— Connie K. Pombo —

Regeneration

My left thigh is shrinking. I see a new hollow place where it used to be round and strong—or stronger. But the muscular dystrophy has snuck in, shot through my body like an octopus's black ink, and started its cruel attack.

I panic every time this happens. I see a slideshow of my worst-case scenario: myself in a wheelchair, dependent on everyone around me, separated from the world by a flight of stairs I can't climb.

I don't ever feel the weakness approaching. I just look down at my body one day and see soft sunken skin, that of an old woman in a hospital bed with flabby flesh hanging from her bones. I noticed it in my right calf for the first time seven years ago. I know there is muscle loss all over my body in random spots, but I can't see my own bony back or the lack of firmness in my butt unless I twist into convoluted positions and stare into my full-length mirror. However, when I sit in the bathtub, knees bent, head resting on an inflatable pillow, there is no ignoring that my left thigh now looks nearly half the size of my right.

Thirty-four years ago when I was diagnosed with FSH muscular dystrophy at age thirteen, I was introduced to the word "degenerative." Every doctor I met told me this was the nature of the disease. Every muscular dystrophy brochure used the word. Even when my neurologist said enthusiastically, "You're doing great. You are degenerating at the speed of a glacier," there was always the understanding that loss of muscle would take place—it was just a matter of how much or how little. I always knew that to some degree my future body would be weaker than the present one.

For most of my life I have hated my body. It has let me down, taken away my ability to play tennis, go for long walks in the woods, carry a heavy bag of groceries. My body is disappearing on me—so slowly and subtly that I have been lulled into trusting its veneer of strength. I sometimes forget it is filled with invaders ready to attack whenever they see a moment of weakness, whenever they carry out a battle plan I don't understand.

Lately, though, something has shifted. I don't despise my body. I no longer curse its awkward gait or look with disgust at my thin right arm. I don't apologize for a physique that is less physically beautiful than it would have been without muscular dystrophy. Instead, I hate the disease. I hate the misguided group of cells or genetic imprint or chromosomal mishap that beats down my body. I hate that it lives with me. I tell it to leave.

I look at my thigh now and speak to it as if it were a child: "Oh, sweetie, I'm so sorry this is happening to you." I pour vanilla-scented massage oil into my palms and tenderly touch the sunken places of my body, sending them all my warmth. I pet my thigh with the same soft gesture I use on Lucy, the fluffy black cat I adore. I gather all the memories of love I have stored inside—the way I ooze with affection when I spend time with my nieces, the way I feel looking into the eyes of a lover—and I pour them onto myself.

A few years ago, I had abdominal surgery. I prepared for it by listening to a meditation tape my mother gave me. A kind woman's voice led me through a series of relaxation techniques. I was guided through every part of my body, slowly softening the places from my head to my fingertips and toes. I imagined myself in my ideal place of relaxation—sometimes staring at the ocean, sometimes lying on a hammock looking up at a sky full of autumn leaves. I visualized my healing taking place.

This was easy to do when I prepared for surgery. I imagined my sweet, skilled surgeon smiling down at me as I lay asleep on the operating table. I imagined all the people praying for me to recover. I said goodbye to my ovary that was to be removed and thanked it for all it had done for me. I imagined waking up easily from my anesthesia, feeling no pain.

I listened to this tape three times a day right up to the moment I was wheeled into surgery. And, as I had seen in my mind's eye, everything went perfectly.

As I recovered at home, I watched in awe as my body began to heal. I had only associated my body with degeneration, but here it was, mending. Initially, I was unable to lie down in bed or sit very long in a chair because of the pain. My stomach was bloated. My incisions were tender and pink. I needed two canes to walk across the room. But every morning I awoke amazed at how much better I felt than the previous day.

I continued to listen to my visualization tape and envision

changes taking place in my body. I saw all my beautiful, wise cells going in to repair the damage like a parade of white-uniformed nurses caring for a patient. I felt each breath bring in fresh air, circulation, and comfort. And then I imagined the next stage of my health: me full of energy sitting in a restaurant with my friends, laughing and sharing food.

After a couple of months I was back to "normal." I was walking with my usual limp but without the canes. I could sleep in bed without wincing, and my stitches disappeared. But I keep playing that visualization tape.

Now, I imagine regeneration because I've seen it can be done. Instead of surgery scenarios, I lie down in the afternoon, close my eyes, and watch as all my muscles get larger and stronger. They intertwine like fingers until they are thick and solid. I envision a large, metal strainer going down my body removing all the specks of dirty, black disease. Then, I picture myself walking easily on a path by the ocean. I am talking with a friend and not even paying attention to each step I take. Sometimes I turn around and walk backwards as we chat, or I skip like I did as a kid. It is so easy, so effortless I feel it in my roots, down to my core. And as the tape ends, I wake up happy and rejuvenated.

I know my body has the ability to heal itself. I know my muscular dystrophy can be cured. I know this as surely as I know my body is deteriorating and there is nothing I can do. Somehow I can hold onto the paradox, knowing that both of these things are true. I never say my hopeful words out loud because everyone knows that muscular dystrophy is degenerative.

I see it in my shrinking thigh. I feel the weariness in my right arm. And yet, when I close my eyes there is a place just as real where I am as fluid as I want to be. There is a place where my body is whole.

~ Karen Myers ~

Brain Strategies for Robust Living

Introduction

A woman named Christine recently called me after hearing about CBT in the break room at work. Her colleague had been discussing different brain tricks she uses to effectively manage anxiety and panic attacks. Christine, not unlike many other first-time callers, introduced herself and asked about learning some of the tricks she'd heard about.

Unfortunately, cognitive behavioral therapy is sometimes misunderstood as being a set of tricks. Cognitive behavioral psychology is *strategic*. It's not magic, nor is it smoke and mirrors. Christine said while she didn't suffer from anxiety like her colleague, she did understand cognitive behavioral psychology could be helpful in managing different emotions when giving speeches or making presentations in public settings. That's what she was hoping to improve. As we wrapped up our phone conversation, I explained that CBT could likely be useful in the areas she wanted, but it would take some effort.

There are a few cognitive behavioral techniques that everyone should know. In fact, some people use them without knowing it. Such techniques can be useful to athletes, business people, or those wanting to maintain positive health and wellness. I'd like to explain some basic, research-based strategies so you can load up your mental health toolbox. Remember, your brain is your body's most important ally. As you read, you will become more knowledgeable about how to effectively use cognitive behavioral tactics, as well as increase the accuracy of your perception of yourself and your health.

Goal Setting for Good Health

First, goal setting is fundamental to understanding how your brain works and also helps focus mental work to make it productive. Unfortunately, many people who attempt to reach long-term goals never identify specific markers that guide them in the direction they're trying to go. You may have time on your side when considering your health goals, or you may be in the same boat as John Buentello who experienced aortic dissection and needed to respond to a new way of living right away. Regardless of timing, goal setting is key to experiencing good health and making changes for the better.

An easy way to remember how to set a good goal is to describe a particular behavior that someone else can see as well. Keep in mind it's not easy to see feelings and emotions, but it is easy to see yourself accomplishing tasks that will promote good health. For example, one good goal would be to eat breakfast seven times a week. As we know, breakfast is the most important meal of the day and studies have proven that skipping it can lead to obesity, not to mention that insufficient fueling can result in decreased concentration at work or school. A problematic goal would be simply to eat breakfast more than you do already. You could do this—eat breakfast more often—but you wouldn't have a good way of tracking the change or knowing exactly when you've met your goal.

Make sure goals are measurable, specific, and concrete. And that means others should be able to observe you reaching them. After you define your personal goals, share them with other people, review them frequently, and adjust them whenever you need to. Write down your goals. Feel free to try it out in the margin of the page right now if you'd like. As you read through the following pages of this chapter, take notes and write down ideas about how to set and reach health-focused goals. Taking time to train your brain is an investment in yourself and in healthy living. Once you have set clear, solid goals then you can move on to using other brain strategies to help you reach them. One of those strategies is positive self-talk.

A Voice You Should Be Hearing

Self-talk is that little voice in your head. And you certainly know that voice can have a positive or negative tone. Research continues to tell us hands-down that you need to develop a positive tone in order to affect your health in a constructive way. When first learning about self-talk, some of my clients laugh and say it seems funny that they are talking to themselves at all. I assure them that it is okay to talk to themselves. It is even okay to answer themselves. I tell them that I do get concerned, however, when they start arguing with themselves, and we usually have a good laugh over that comment.

Positive self-talk is using your inner voice and self-instruction to advise yourself. Sometimes we need to be coached away from that dessert on the menu, or be encouraged to run that one last mile on the treadmill. For some people, the voice in their heads can be awfully critical. It can be helpful to track your thoughts over a period of time. For example, you may want to record your particular thoughts when you have negative emotions. Keeping a thought log is a spectacular idea for recognizing negative themes or trends in your thinking. And once you identify those trends, you may be able to change and restructure your thinking as we discussed in previous chapters.

Do You See What I See?

Along with positive self-talk, add visualization to your psychological armamentarium. A remarkable article written by Barbel Knauper and colleagues at McGill University appeared in *Psychology & Health* in 2011. It describes the benefit of visualization and how it is useful when trying to increase healthy food selection habits. Researchers asked participants to devise a plan for eating more fruit in their diets. They also asked participants to visualize how the plan would be implemented. For example, participants in the study might have seen themselves shopping for, washing, and putting fruit into salads, not to mention packing it for lunch or taking it along as a snack on weekend outings. Fruit consumption doubled when planning and visualization were part of the participants' food habits. This research showcases a perfect example of a basic mental strategy that can benefit your health.

Imagine this…

Visualize biting into an unpeeled orange. Feel the texture of the rind, the cool temperature of the rind against your teeth, the pressure of your teeth pushing through the rind, tasting the bitter, and then feeling and tasting the flavorful juice explode in your mouth. Now, if you want to see how well you visualized, grab an orange and take a bite!

Over the years I have come to see the incredible value of visualization. Visualization, sometimes called imagery, is a fantastic way of letting your brain experience something new, or corrective, without having to go through an actual physical action. I have seen people rid themselves of phobias, learn to do brand new tasks, and become more consistent in specific behaviors, like anger management or interacting successfully with co-workers or new friends. To illustrate what I mean, let me tell you a quick story about someone I'll call Paul.

For no clear, identifiable reason Paul had developed a phobia that was quite unusual. Paul was afraid of umbrellas. It's okay, go ahead and laugh. Paul did as well, as long as he wasn't around an umbrella! Using visualization, Paul was able to eliminate some of the fears he had. Paul responded well to a behavioral technique called systematic desensitization, which is a combination of relaxation strategies and deliberate exposure to a fearful stimulus ranked in a hierarchy from lowest fear to highest fear. We started by imagining umbrellas in the distance, then umbrellas up close and, finally, interacting with an umbrella, opening and closing it. For Paul's desensitization, visualization was the key. I could explain more about the effectiveness of desensitization for Paul, but for now I'd like to describe how visualization was helpful to him and what you can learn from his umbrella phobia.

Paul did an exceptional job of using all of his senses when he visualized umbrellas. That means that he did not just see an umbrella but he was able to feel its plastic handle. He was able to feel the rain on a wet umbrella. He could smell the nylon fabric. He even pushed himself to hear the umbrella as the automatic opener clicked and the ribs popped open, creating a small puff of damp, musty air. You get the picture. Once Paul was able to use visualization and relaxation to reduce his fears, he also learned visualization was helpful in other areas of his life, such as improving his skills while skiing, weightlifting, and taking ballroom dancing lessons with his wife.

You can use visualization to help keep your health strong, too. As the Boston Marathon medical team psychologist, I've found that many of the runners I've worked with often visualize themselves running well, rather than struggling, in the later miles of the marathon. Visualization can also be helpful in physical rehabilitation after an injury, smoking cessation, weight management, preparation for surgical procedures, and breast-feeding. When you use visualization to practice new or corrective behaviors, however, be sure to practice them in real time. That means visualize at the same pace or speed an activity or behavior would actually occur. When done correctly, visualization is an extraordinary way of letting your brain experience life without having to actually be in a specific situation physically.

Association and Dissociation: A Useful Pair

Have you ever had the experience of driving down the highway and finding that your mind is focused on something else important while you are continuing to drive? Where did the miles go? Highway hypnosis is a common occurrence most drivers identify with. It's also a fine example of how dissociation happens. First, though, you need to know how dissociation differs from its counterpart, association.

Think of association and dissociation somewhat like siblings who are almost nothing alike, but are still related by attention. On one hand, association is a strategy that pairs your experience with some other object, so you can complete a task. For example, if you are trying to finish a 5K run and are struggling to work your way to the finish line, you may want to think of yourself as a locomotive gaining steam and momentum, pushing toward the station. You draw on the power and strength of the locomotive that you associate with.

Dissociation, on the other hand, happens when you take your mind off the present and put it onto something that is unrelated to your immediate physical experience, particularly when that experience is painful. Take that last push toward the 5K finish, for instance. You have a side stitch, your mouth is dry, and you're convinced you have matching blisters on your ankles from your new running shoes. Instead of focusing on those details, you start to dissociate by casting your attention toward a much more enjoyable image or activity you concoct in your mind. You may think about the details of a Mexican dinner you are planning for next weekend at your house, or perhaps you'd rather think about relaxing in a jute-braided hammock, waiting for an enormous fish to grab the bait and spin the reel on your never-miss fishing rod.

Dissociation is a very effective strategy, but any discussion about it should also include a warning: pain has an important function for your body and that's to tell you something's not right. Pain should always be addressed, and evaluated by a medical professional. You should never push through pain if you don't know exactly what its origin is.

With that disclaimer stated, dissociation can be a great brain strategy for managing uncomfortable emotional or physical aspects of living. For example, if you have to get a weekly shot for allergies or have another uncomfortable procedure related to healthcare, dissociation can be helpful if the pain is difficult or intolerable.

Try this real-life example. Pinch your arm. Make the pinch painful to the degree of about seven on a scale of 1 to 10. Be sure not to hurt yourself. Now keep that pain at level seven but toss your mind onto something else like a favorite dessert.

Think about the dessert and its flavors, its textures, its temperature, its appearance when you first see it. Just hold that image in your mind. Now stop and reevaluate the level of the pain in your arm on that same scale of 1 to 10. Has your level changed from a seven? Most people find while imaging the dessert the pain level noticeably decreased. Why? It's nearly impossible to tune into the pain and the favorite dessert at same time. If you notice what I am describing, then you have successfully used dissociation. Again, remember that dissociation should be used only after you know for certain that the pain you experience is not your body's way of telling you that something's wrong.

There are many other effective brain strategies that can be used to enhance life and health. You've just read about some of the more popular ones that can be immediately helpful. Try these strategies whenever you get a chance. Practice will almost make perfect.

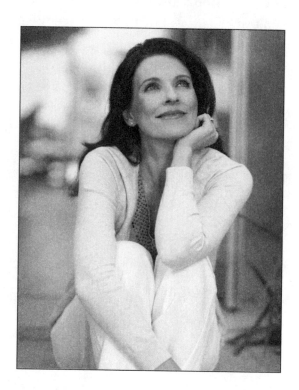

Chapter 6
Increase Your Health IQ — Now!

Spying on the Enemy

I n 2006 I began a journey through the U.S. healthcare system that to this moment has not ended. In April of that year I began walking very strangely. I couldn't walk in a straight line without bumping into the wall. It was as if my "steering" was off. So I went to the doctor and the first question posed to a young person with such a problem is: when was the last time you drank alcohol or took drugs? Since I don't drink alcohol, nor do I take drugs, they were at a loss. No one really had a clue as to what the problem was, and finally they said perhaps it was just an ear infection. I was given medication to combat dizziness and was sent on my merry way. In October of that year one side of my entire head went numb; this led to an MRI, which led to the discovery of lesions in my brain.

"What could cause lesions?" I asked very innocently.

"Multiple sclerosis" was the reply.

After I hung up the phone, I began to bawl my eyes out. I didn't know anything about multiple sclerosis except for one thing: one of my adopted uncles had it, and by this time he was using a scooter to move around. I thought perhaps I only had a week or so left to walk, and I too would soon be in a scooter. I didn't know what to do with myself. I called my sister and she told me to do one thing—"pray." And so I prayed, and a calm came over me. Now I would love to tell you that after that moment every test I ever took again showed no MS, but I can't. I do have multiple sclerosis.

It wasn't the easiest thing to accept, but I found that for me, knowledge was power. I signed up with my local MS society to receive literature—the initial series they sent was called "Knowledge Is Power." I knew then I was on the right track. I read about the illness, I joined an MS forum to observe how other people with MS coped. I was also able to talk to those who were going through similar experiences, and finally I set about getting familiar with my "new normal."

I started to realize that the reason I had such a complete breakdown that first day was because I knew nothing about MS. When I began to learn more about it, I felt as if I was part of a covert operation, snooping on this illness that was now my body's enemy. The more I learned about it, the more equipped I felt to make the decisions that I needed in order to conduct my life.

Now don't get me wrong, learning about MS was no treat. At some points I wished I still did not know what I had, only because the future can look quite bleak for those of us who have this illness. I sat myself down and decided to look at it this way: Yes, I have this crummy disease. No I don't have a life like my friends do, and sometimes I get sad about that—but I'm not them, I'm me. This is my life and when I wake up in the morning, with the ability to move and exercise, that's a reason to be happy. Do I worry? Yes! I do because I'm human, and this disease causes loss of mobility. I worry about losing my eyesight, and my ability to walk one day, but I pray it won't snatch my smile now or then for that matter. Do I feel awful sometimes? Uh, yes! That's the nature of illness, but it doesn't mean I can't be kind to you or give you an encouraging word.

Sometimes, doctors seem to think I don't understand the scope of my health issues, but they're the ones who do not understand the scope of my faith. If you see your options, pray for guidance to choose the right option, and then make the decision to go forward as long as you possibly can, people will have a difficult time getting in your way.

Will you be happy-go-lucky all the time? Perhaps not, but you will keep on moving forward; you won't get stuck in a mindset that can hold you hostage to negative thoughts and attitudes.

Can I do everything that I was once able to? No, but I value the things I still can do, and count my blessings as often as I can. I also realized and was grateful that there are some things that I can do now that I couldn't do before!

Someone might say that positive thinking couldn't possibly have such an effect, but I think it does. My last MRI was a little shocking to my doctor; she even said, "Looking at this MRI, I wouldn't think that you are the person it belonged to."

I am able to do this, I believe, partly due to my belief in God and partly due to having the wonderful mother I did. My mother had lupus, which destroyed her kidneys. She was on dialysis for about ten years before she died, yet she conducted her life with such grace and gratitude that it still awes me today. I have a hard time not doing my best to follow her example.

Throughout my time dealing with MS I have been able to write an article for a national MS magazine, and start a small blog about MS to educate and encourage younger people battling the disease. Learning more about my illness is one of the things that helped me keep my attitude in check and made me feel most like myself again. My tactic might not work for every single other person who has MS or will ever be diagnosed with it, but I don't want to hide what worked for me—just in case it is able to help someone else.

~ Maxine Young ~

A Change of Mind

Shock. Disbelief. Despair.

My gynecologist had given me the result of several tests... ovarian cancer.

Within a week, extensive exploratory surgery told the awful truth. The cancer had already progressed to Stage IIIC, advanced disease. The odds for my survival were bleak.

Eight rounds of chemotherapy followed, taking their toll on my body and emotions. Discouragement, distress, and anxiety arrived and settled in for an extended stay.

I discovered a common experience shared with every cancer patient I talked with—at least one traumatic event had preceded our illnesses. In my case, the deaths of close family members plus highly stressful situations at my workplace left me reeling. Unearthing and dealing with the thoughts and emotions that accompanied these incidents became my top priority. What I found buried deep within was ugly—anger, resentment, depression, and broken dreams.

This happened nearly sixteen years ago. How did I cope and survive?

Along with adopting a healthier diet, I finally recognized that many of my thought patterns had been extremely negative. Through various books, seminars, and workshops, I learned that thoughts are powerful "things" which may adversely affect our health, but can be revised and controlled to improve wellbeing.

I certainly had a compelling incentive—life!

During the period of transforming my thoughts from harmful to healthy thinking, I began to stop and really feel how my body reacted when negative attitudes and emotions were present. My blood pressure rose, muscles automatically tightened, breathing became shallow—all normal responses from the sympathetic nervous system preparing my body to battle any perceived predators. However, because I'd allowed myself to stay in this perpetual state of fight or flight, it had resulted in a great strain on my body.

The main culprit for me was lack of forgiveness. I had remained in that prison cell far too long. At last, I understood by continually replaying hurtful events in my mind, rehearsing what I'd like to say to "tell them off," and fantasizing about revenge, I'd actually handed over control of my life to those I had not forgiven.

I decided on a change of mind when I realized that not forgiving is like drinking poison—it only hurts the one who consumes it. True, a price still had to be paid by the offenders; however, it wasn't my responsibility to enact judgment. God would take care of that.

Sometimes, modern medicine overlooks the prominent role our minds play in overall health. No prescription medication can change a destructive lifestyle or mindset. A brief look at the tragic lives of many singers, actors, and athletes shows that money and privilege can't buy happiness or contentment. Focusing on things that are true, honorable, and positive goes a long way toward healing.

By God's mercy, I overcame the grim survival predictions for my type of cancer. Through prayer and a changed state of mind, I'm in great health and thriving. I've learned to forgive myself and others quickly so anger and resentment cannot pollute my mind and body.

Forgiveness started with an intentional decision of will, for my own health's sake. A change of mind was the greatest gift I could ever give myself—it transformed my life.

— Ann Holbrook —

A Gentle Touch
Works Wonders

I grew up in the Northern California lumber town of Scotia, where the streets were full of holes, the driveways were gravel, and the drab little company homes were lined up in tight rows. The people who lived there were as austere as the town itself. They were wiry timber fallers, grizzled green-chain pullers and women who were constructed of hardship and despair. These were salt-of-the-earth folks locked in a never-ending struggle to make ends meet.

I was taught at a young age that strength equaled survival and that men should never show emotion. Any sign of affection was thought of as a weakness. Hugging was considered girly behavior. Crying was expressly forbidden.

Scotia was a cold, impersonal place to grow up, but one moment stands out in my childhood like a beacon of light. It happened in the fourth grade when a classmate and I were sitting in the playground at recess. My friend picked a dandelion and twirled it around my face (a test to see if I liked girls, I think). It was an unexpected moment of tenderness, a delightful experience that completely surprised me. It also would have spelled disaster if anyone had seen us.

Still, I felt transformed. That gentle moment had a big impact on me. As one who was raised to fear touch, I came to realize that human contact was fundamental to health and happiness. More than fifty years later I'm even more convinced. Touch is a basic need of babies, adolescents, adults and the elderly. It's one way that we seem designed to communicate.

Touch has elicited much interest over the past few decades. Research shows that what has been called "therapeutic touch" has many positive effects on children and on people who suffer from various illnesses. Touch promotes healthy development, enhances the body's ability to self-regulate, and even helps us control our emotions.

Animals require touch, too. It forms an essential part of their interactions, especially between mother and baby. Touch sensations in rats, for example, are absolutely necessary for the survival of the pups. If a mother rat doesn't lick her newborns they will die. The touch sensation of licking promotes the release of digestive hormones necessary for the pups to use in processing food.

Human babies also need and seek the experience of touch. All mammals, including whales, are massaged immediately upon birth. Many infant mammals (including all primates) sleep close to their mother and become distressed if they do not have body contact. The human infant is programmed with a number of reflexes to recognize the mother at birth and to stay beside her.

Children of preschool age need a large supply of touch experiences. If you've ever watched toddlers or preschoolers in a playground setting, you've probably noticed that there are a lot of touch exchanges between them. They embrace each other, wrestle, and push one another in a playful way. They also periodically seek out their teachers for contact, to embrace them or just to feel their closeness from time to time. Most toddlers need to be held periodically to "gather their strength," emotionally speaking, which enables them to continue their explorations.

Touch has many other useful purposes, especially for adults. It calms the heart, relieves tension and relaxes muscles. Touch can even alter temperament and attitude.

My kids were taught from a young age to touch and hug. It was a lesson my wife and I instilled in them. I've been widowed now for seven years. The children are almost grown and most of my time is spent alone. I've slogged through the years feeling depressed but not really understanding why. One night, after a late dinner in a restaurant, the waitress stood chatting with me. When she handed me the bill, she placed her hand on my shoulder, patting it affectionately. I paid and left. Out in my pickup I burst into tears, finally understanding the reason for my depression: I had been starved for human contact. I hadn't felt the gentle touch of another person in years.

Things are much different today. Now I happily touch everyone I encounter (who I sense will not reject it). I also gladly give out hugs. After all, no one should ever go without a daily dose of love and tenderness. It's the touch of a gentle hand that our souls crave.

~ Timothy Martin ~

Running
with a Smile

For more than forty years, I've been running for exercise. Three or four miles, three or four times a week. And hating every step.

So when I learned about the Tarahumara Indians, who live in Mexico's remote Copper Canyons and are renowned for running long distances wearing little more than homemade sandals and a smile, I was intrigued. Fascinated. Amazed.

Not just that they run hundreds of miles with only worn tire rubber tied to their feet, but that they smile while doing it. Why? Because the Tarahumara know something most other runners don't: Running is supposed to be fun. Not torture. Not penance for eating an extra-large piece of apple pie with two scoops of vanilla ice cream. Not something you do to keep your skinny jeans from getting too tight or because you might get a medal at the end of a race.

For thousands of years, the Tarahumara have excelled at combining breath and mind and muscle into seemingly effortless movement over some of the most rugged terrain on earth. Simply because they understand what it means to love running.

Could a slightly overweight middle-aged woman (me, for instance) learn to love it, too?

I didn't trade my hundred-dollar running shoes with the

cushioned heels and high-tech pronation control orthotics for flip-flops. But I did buy a pair of flexible shoes with a low heel-to-toe differential, hoping they would encourage me to run with a more natural gait. I replaced the junk food in my diet with real food. Carrots instead of Cheetos. Oranges instead of Oreos. Peas instead of pizza. And I added a couple of spoonfuls of chia seeds, which the Tarahumara swear provide an unbeatable energy boost, to my daily regimen.

Last but not least, I vowed to smile every time I ran.

Smiling felt a little silly at first. But after a while, I noticed that many of the drivers I encountered on my running route smiled back at me. Some waved. A few tooted their horns. I began to pay attention to scenery I'd come to take for granted. A newborn calf hiding behind her mother. A great blue heron admiring his reflection in a pond. A fencerow alive with black-eyed Susans and Queen Anne's lace.

It wasn't long before I quit dreading my runs. Soon, I actually began to enjoy them. Now when I lace up my new low-tech running shoes and head out the door, I rarely have to remind myself that running is supposed to be fun. I won't pretend that I smile for the entire three or four miles. I tend to grimace on the curves and groan on the uphills. But whenever I hit a shady spot or encounter an unexpected cool breeze or kick it into high gear on the downhill home stretch, I don't just smile. I grin.

Just like the Tarahumara who inspired me.

~ Jennie Ivey ~

Increase Your
Health IQ—Now!

Introduction

An epiphany. Realization. An "aha" moment. Regardless of what you call it; insight is gained in that split-second when you go from not knowing something to knowing it. It's a remarkable feeling, actually. Some people even report that they feel their brain physically shift when they gain new, powerful information or develop an informed perspective. While the brain has an enormous capacity to change (which is called neuroplasticity), I am certain major cerebral structures aren't swapping physical positions like an odd game of musical chairs. Your brain can, however, assimilate new information quickly. It is whirring along at an incredible, efficient speed.

When you gain insight, you are coming face to face with life-changing information. When considering the relationship between your brain and great health, research reveals a lot about the personality traits, social connections, healthy thinking, and other psychological processes that are at play in your head. By gathering information about current research trends and learning how your psychological self interrelates to health, you can experience motivating aha moments, as well as influence thinking for positive health for both yourself and even your family. To increase your health IQ, read on.

Smile and Feel the Difference!

In a 2009 *Time* magazine article, journalist John Cloud reflected on his trainer's recommendation to keep a neutral face rather than grimacing when working out strenuously at the gym. Cloud's article, which includes a photo of Stevie Wonder's unmistakable broad grin, ties together age-old theory and contemporary research about the influence facial expressions have on emotions. Most research concludes that your outward facial expression *does* tell the world how you're feeling on the inside.

An article in the *Journal of Personality and Social Psychology*, written by David Matsumoto of San Francisco State University and Bob Willingham of the Center for Psychological Studies in Berkeley, California, examined real and social emotions felt in sighted and non-sighted individuals. For the sake of definition in this case, real emotions are those feelings that are genuine and authentic and occur as a result of an event that would typically prompt them. Social emotions, in contrast, are emotions or expressions that occur in order for social interactions to be successful. Matsumoto and Willingham concluded that sighted and non-sighted people both express facial expressions equally.

However, since blind individuals have never had the advantage of visually observing others' expressions, it's convincing that their faces are truly reflective of actual emotions and vice versa. So, when you're feeling glum, irritable, or peeved, try smiling away the negative emotion you're feeling on the inside. When you reduce negative emotions and replace them with positive ones, you'll be realigning yourself with the emotional characteristics of healthy thinkers. It appears to me that's exactly what

Jennie Ivey does when she's running and racking up mileage on her smile. And of course, becoming a healthy thinker translates to healthier living. Now that's something you can smile about!

Dangle a Carrot... or Green Bean... or Broccoli

Unless you are disconnected from the world of nutrition, you know about the importance of vegetables in the human diet. Without doing almost anything else, you can make immediate positive health changes simply by eating vegetables throughout your day. The U.S. Department of Agriculture asserts that eating plenty of vegetables not only provides your body with the healthy nutrients it needs, but also helps combat chronic diseases such as Type II diabetes and obesity, and reduces the chance of stroke and some types of cancer. Once you get into the habit, eating veggies can become as routine as reading the morning paper, checking e-mail, or brushing your teeth. But if you do commit to adding more leafy greens to your daily diet, it'll be easier if you get the entire family involved. Don't go it alone!

Researchers at the University of Granada offer helpful insight into how to make a dinner table overhaul. Children, particularly those six and under, are apt to eat up to 80 percent more vegetables if they're allowed to choose the ones they want to eat. The Spanish researchers tell us that while some younger children may not like certain vegetables because of the bitter flavor, which may be especially strong to younger palates, overall vegetable consumption still increased. So when you are shifting gears at the dinner table, be sure to include a variety of both familiar and new options. Talk with your family about what veggies they'd like to see on the table, making sure they have a choice in the matter. You may also want to include family members on grocery store outings, trips to the local farmers' market, or even to the bookstore to help find interesting recipes for healthier meals. Making a game of trying new or unusual vegetables (we call it "Try a Bite" at our house) can be a hilarious and healthy way to successfully get more healthy foods on your family dinner table. Following is a table of healthy and interesting foods that may help jumpstart your dinner table overhaul.

Extraordinarily Healthy and Entertaining Foods for Kids to Try

Food	Benefit
The Ugli Fruit	Vitamin C
Dragon Fruit	Antioxidants
Sea Beans	Naturally salty
White Asparagus	Vitamins A & C, Fiber
Edamame	Protein and Fiber

Serve a Family Meal Tonight—
and at Least Two More This Week

A 2011 journal article in *Pediatrics* chewed on the importance of eating family meals together with teenagers. The research concluded that teenagers positively benefited from eating at least three family meals together each week. Not only did teenagers eat more nutritiously *en famille*, but those who ate at least three meals were less apt to be overweight and also independently chose healthy foods. This morsel of research also indicated teenagers truly enjoy being part of the family meal experience, as long as they feel like they are respected and have a voice at the table.

The benefits of eating together as a family are twofold. First, teenagers gain both nutritionally and socially, battling early childhood diabetes and obesity while attempting to set healthy eating habits. Secondly, adults sitting at a table with teenagers can gain an advantage of being connected to family, exchanging positive emotions, teaching reciprocal communication, and family values.

Lung Darts and Healthy Living Don't Mix

Stopping smoking should be a no-brainer when it comes to improving your health. Yet the Center for Disease Control and Prevention reported in 2009 that there were more than 46 million adult smokers (not including adolescents) in the United States. That means about one in five Americans smoke.

Sure, it is difficult to stop smoking, but the payoff is certainly worth it. At home or overseas, almost every pack of cigarettes displays some sort of warning about how they are detrimental to your health. In some of my recent international travels, I've seen cigarette packages with large, bold imprints that patently state, "Cigarettes will kill you." Other public awareness campaigns aimed at reducing smoking include pictures of cancerous, decaying gums or people dying of lung disease. If you have seen any of these images, you will agree that a picture is worth 1,000 words.

Jean Weiss, an MSN health and fitness writer, superbly highlighted the immediate health benefits that come from choosing not to smoke. You'll review them very soon. First, though, Weiss cited Deputy Chief Medical Officer of the American Cancer Society Len Lichtenfeld, MD, who indicated that just over a third of smokers tried to quit in 2009, but only 10 to 20 percent of them remained successful three months after quitting. It's a challenge to quit smoking, but the benefits are almost immediate. If you are a smoker, or know someone who smokes, read through the following table and see how health can improve by maintaining a cigarette-free lifestyle. Even if you've tried to quit before and failed, don't get discouraged — you're in good company. Sources agree that quitting smoking is something most people will fail at a few times before they succeed. So, keep trying! Read on for some great incentives for snuffing out something that's certainly killing you.

Stop Time	Health Benefit
20 minutes after quitting	Heart rate and blood pressure will drop
12 hours after quitting	Carbon monoxide level in your blood falls to normal
2-3 weeks after quitting	Functioning in circulation and lungs improve
9 months after quitting	Reduction in coughing and/or shortness of breath
1 year after quitting	Coronary heart disease risk drops to half compared to when you were smoking
5 years after quitting	Your risk for a stroke is the same as if you'd never smoked

10 years after quitting	Your chances of dying of lung cancer are half of what they would have been as a smoker. Your risk of various cancers, including bladder, mouth, throat, cervix and pancreas have decreased.
15 years after quitting	Coronary heart disease risk is the same as if you had never smoked

Loosen the Grip on Negative Feelings

Remember defense mechanisms in Chapter 2? We gave credit to Sigmund Freud for identifying and naming those psychological processes. We can also thank Freud for the well-known psychological maxim: "Depression is anger turned inward."

In my experience working with clients, this phrase proves to be true. There are a multitude of reasons why we may be angry at people, at ourselves, or about situations and outcomes. But it's not necessarily the origin of our anger that matters as much as what we do about it. Dozens of new clients have entered my practice angry over one thing or another but simply haven't done anything to address it. Worse yet, not only had they kept their anger undercover, but they convinced people they were happy in general. Honestly, below the happiness façade was un-resolved negative emotion. I've seen it happen time and again.

Even though it's not a pleasant process, clients who work toward ridding themselves of negative emotions frequently ex-perience an improvement in health and quality of life. Of course, one of the first steps you may have to take is to acknowledge a negative feeling exists and that it may not last forever.

Several years ago, a patient provided a wonderful de-scription for this transformation. She had four kids, had gone through a heated divorce, and was struggling to collect child support from her ex-husband, who was living by a careless and excessive financial standard. While she wanted to appear to her friends and family as though she was dealing well with her life stress, she was not. Instead, she harbored unbearable re-sentment toward her ex-husband, who had had an affair while she was pregnant with twins. Over time, she found therapy to be a place where she could work on her anger and depres-sion. And as her anger and depression began to dissipate, the woman acknowledged that she didn't realize how bad she had been feeling. "You know," she said to me, "even water is begin-ning to taste better to me now."

Research suggests that when we therapeutically address anger, negotiate grudges, or forgive someone, we positively affect our health in many ways. Lowering blood pressure, re-lieving chronic pain, decreasing the likelihood of substance abuse, and increasing healthy relationships are all examples of how health can be affected positively when anger is relieved.

Sizing Them Up Matters

What do you think about the guy who lives down the street? Describe your best friend to me. What are the strengths and weaknesses of the person with whom you work the closest? Before you begin tossing around opinions of others, you need to know that Wake Forest University Assistant Professor Dustin Wood suggests that descriptions of others may reveal more about you than you realize. Professor Wood and his crew believe an individual's tendency to describe others more positively or more negatively may very well reflect levels of positivity and negativity in the life of the evaluator.

You've surely known at least one person in life who's critical of others or whose faultfinding skill surpasses anyone you know. How likely is it that person is happy, content and optimistic? Not very, I'd guess. This built-in gauge is an exceptional new gift you have for gaining insight into how negativity may impair healthy living. If your evaluations of others tend to lean in a negative direction, perhaps you should consider that the lens you're using to view them through needs cleaning. In sum, if your internal world is not satisfying, otherwise healthy relationships can suffer as a result. Working toward emotional balance and remediation of negativity in your personal world can enhance social interactions with others and increase healthy connections.

Your Health Is a Laughing Matter

In the 1970's, journalist and editor Norman Cousins first claimed that belly laughs from Marx Brothers films helped his

cardiac condition. A layperson trying to focus on positive emotions and his health, Cousins set up the idea of humor and
health like a good joke; but, the punch line wasn't a gag. His
claims were legitimate.

So you've heard that laughter is the best medicine? Here's
one reason that old maxim holds some water. In 2009, Michael
Miller, MD and William Fry, MD described a complex connection between laughter and blood flow. Perhaps you could say
that they got to the heart of the matter by considering mirthful
laughter. What is mirthful laughter? It's the type of laughter that
comes from old-fashioned humor, compared to other forms of
laughter used to increase communication or build rapport. All
joking aside, in their earlier work, the University of Maryland
Medical Center at Baltimore researchers suggested that
laughing at least fifteen minutes a day helps improve vascular
system health.

Simple Side-Splitter Strategies

1. Watch funny movies and TV shows
2. Learn, then tell some fresh jokes
3. Download some standup comedy routines on
   your iPod
4. Go to a comedy club with friends
5. Sign up for an improvisation class
6. Increase time with funny friends

To reach this conclusion, Miller and his troop had participants watch both humorous and stressful movies. It turns out that laughing caused the tissues lining blood vessels to expand, thus increasing blood flow, whereas viewing stressful images caused a constriction of the vessels, which reduced blood flow. In some cases, laughter even generated health benefits similar to aerobic exercise. But while a healthy vascular system means improved physical and cognitive functioning, Miller warns that chuckles and giggles should not replace treadmills, elliptical machines, and your favorite walking or running shoes.

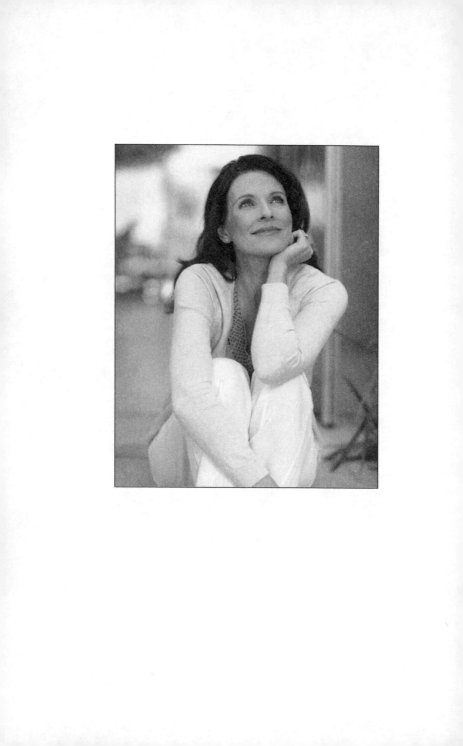

Chapter 7
Avoid the F-word: Frustration

Hypochondria's Awesome... Seriously

At the age of fifteen years and five months, I was diagnosed with high cholesterol. Wait, what? That was my initial reaction too. Let me rewind a little. My family's insanely susceptible to cardiovascular diseases. And I, being the hypochondriac that I am, decided to get a lipid profile done the day I learnt fifteen was the correct age to do so. When I told my mother, she suppressed any incredulous emotions she may have had, and agreed to allow me. I strolled into the pathology lab, paid for a lipid profile and thyroid test, and watched as my blood was collected in a little vial.

Now, I didn't expect anything but normal results. I'm a pretty healthy person. I've been vegetarian since I was six, rarely consume processed food, eat an insane amount of fruits and vegetables, and, while nobody will ever call me a sportswoman, lead a highly non-sedentary lifestyle. That's why, when I got the report back, I didn't expect to see my LDL levels highlighted urgently. While the maximum LDL level (bad cholesterol) for a person should be 100 mg/dL, mine was 107. At my age, it's a terrible, alarming cause of concern.

When I mentioned this to my mother, she snatched the

report from my hand and studied it in shock, unmindful of the fact that she was supposed to have both hands on the steering wheel and eyes on the road ahead of her. Swerving past a sleeping cow and acrobatically avoiding a swearing driver, all she could do was curse.

Of course she knew the implications of this. Now, I won't go into the biological details of high cholesterol at the age of fifteen. However, there's one thing that my family's cardiologist told me: it's genetic. You need to be careful, or it will spiral out of control, and you'll be lying on a hospital bed in twenty years, repenting.

I took drastic measures to bring down my cholesterol levels. I gave up processed food completely, and ate as much as my body needed—not more, not less. I didn't falter for a very long time. Then, all of a sudden, I broke down. I ate the wrong things. I exercised half-heartedly. My grades plummeted, and I snapped at everybody around me. Predictably, my weight ballooned. My cholesterol levels had obviously gone up; however, I never bothered checking them.

One day, I came across a quote by the august Emerson: "Our greatest glory is not in never failing, but in rising up every time we fail." I don't know why that had such a big impact on me. I have read and heard hundreds of wise words by exceptional women and men, yet that quote stayed in my mind.

Soon enough, I rose like a phoenix from the ashes of failure, and reared my head once again. The extra pounds fell off, and my grades picked up again. I managed to control my condition, and I felt wonderful. Of course, I give in to temptations occasionally, but I can control myself now. I know that, ultimately, I'm responsible for myself. My loved ones can try to guide me, but they can't live my life. So, whatever decisions I take have to come from deep within my heart if I'm to succeed. Luckily for me, I learnt that very early in my life.

I'm not infallible. I make mistakes, and I feel my heart skip a terrifying beat every time I do so. But I won't give up. I can't. "But still, like air, I'll rise."

— Supriya Ambwani —

Paddling Away Stress

Droplets of water fall from my paddle as it dips into the lake and emerges. My arm muscles flex as they drive the kayak forward away from the pull of the shore. Under the bright sunlight the lake shimmers like thousands of tiny diamonds. This is fitting because the lake is my treasure.

Lake Arthur at Moraine State Park in western Pennsylvania is my home away from home. The 3,225-acre watery playground is away from the crowds, the traffic and the city that seems to continuously expand as new shopping plazas are constructed.

It's not the place that time forgot, but it's a place where I can forget time and just be. There are no cell phones, no computers and no distractions. I can paddle the lake, exploring its nooks and crannies, or nap in a cove as my kayak bobs in the gentle waves. My clock is the sun and when it starts its journey west, I know it's time to go back to my life. A life I sometimes try to forget.

I was diagnosed with multiple sclerosis, a demyelinating autoimmune disease that affects the central nervous system, a year ago. As the doctor's words sealed my fate I wondered if activities like kayaking would even be possible.

MS is like a glue that I can't get off my body. There is always something: tingling in the feet, fatigue, itchiness, brain fog. There's no cure and I can feel great one day and half alive the next. It affects my work life, making me forget how to do things, and my home life, by overwhelming me with fatigue.

There is only one place where I can seem to escape MS—the lake. I don't know if it's the exertion of paddling that chases the fatigue away, the sunlight that doses my body with vitamin D or the oneness with nature that quiets my soul, but on the lake I am stress-free and I can leave all my worries on the shore.

Fluffy white clouds drift above as I paddle away from shore. A blue heron is perched on a partially submerged trunk of a fallen tree and I head towards it. I lay my paddle across my boat and let my orange kayak glide through the water so as not to startle the bird.

It's so peaceful on the lake and everything feels right in the world. I've seen birds perform the most amazing aeronautic feats. I've sat just off shore and watched a doe and her two fawns come down to the water's edge and drink. I've seen baby animals play, blissfully unaware that a human is even nearby.

After my diagnosis I started treatment and began the long arduous journey of healing myself. I credit kayaking as one of the reasons I'm doing so well with the disease. The lake provides the escape I need from needles, nurses and the constant reminder that I live with a chronic disease. Whenever I'm paddling against the waves or cruising with the current I'm reminded that life is worth fighting for.

~ Valerie D. Benko ~

No One Wins the Blame Game

"I'm sorry to tell you this, but it appears you're having a miscarriage." Through the phone I could feel the night nurse's compassion, but she couldn't do anything more for me than to describe what my body would endure over the next few hours. Sadly, she was right. Our first baby's journey, after twelve weeks of what seemed to be a very healthy pregnancy, was coming to an abrupt end.

No drinking. No smoking. Prenatal vitamins. Regular checkups. I thought I was doing everything right to provide a healthy and nourishing body for my unborn child. So many questions, but they would remain unanswered for a while as I desperately tried to deal with the emotional and physical pain at hand. We called family members at 2 a.m. to ask for prayers for my peace as I started down a long night of pain and tears.

In the final hour of the most disheartening day of my life, I lay in a small hospital room with my obstetrician and my husband by my side. All hopes of my baby's survival had passed. All they could do was to comfort me. And all I could focus on was the feel of the textured wallpaper as I repeatedly ran my fingertips over the wall. I didn't hear a word they said. I don't even think I could feel their touch. Everything in that room at that very moment became very distant and surreal.

The ride home was quiet. Jeff held my hand and twirled my wedding band as we drove. I sat in silence, wondering if he blamed me for the day's events. Over the course of the next few days, multiple times he told me that wasn't the case—that sometimes these things happen. He seemed to understand the natural selection process much better than I did. He was sad—I could see it. He shed tears while packing up the few newborn gifts we had, but his pain, as he tells it, was completely different from mine. He hurt for me, and the pain I felt; and for some reason, he was filled with hope—hope that we would again conceive and start our family.

I, on the other hand, was a world apart from feeling those emotions.

Unable to shake the "blame game," I began a rapid decline to what might have been diagnosed as depression had I taken the steps to see a doctor. Instead, I found that wadding my feelings up in a ball was more comfortable. And, if those feelings weren't filling enough, I would eat. Sugar. Carbs. Whatever. If my body couldn't be filled with a child that I knew I would love and cherish, then surely food must be able to take its place. Three months of stress eating, eleven extra pounds on my hips, and barely a smile from my usually cheery face were becoming a combination for disaster. Family and friends suggested a counselor, but I objected. I didn't have a problem. I lost a baby, but I wasn't crazy—and I certainly could do this alone without the help of a stranger.

A couple more months, several more pounds, and an insane belief that I had somehow caused the termination of my pregnancy ultimately led me to make an appointment with my family practitioner. I went to the appointment expecting her to be on my side, telling me what I wanted to hear, but instead she harshly stated the cold facts. "Heidi, this stress is sending you into depression and you need to take care of this." I held up my hand, hoping to stop her from talking, but she continued. "There are prescription drugs that will help. Or, I can suggest a counselor." I shut my eyes, shook my head and held my hand up higher.

"I don't take pills, and I will not talk to a counselor." I adamantly repeated the words until she laid an ultimatum on the table. "I'm not letting you go out that door until you choose one. You need help. Choose one." Smugly, I chose the easy way out. "Fine. Give me the pills." To humor her, I filled the prescription on the way home. Two hours later, I emptied the entire bottle in the toilet. Ha! I showed her!

Two weeks later a co-worker shared her story of miscarriage, and I was surprised to see her smiling during our conversation. After months of dealing with her own loss, she was not dead inside. She was hopeful. She had a joy that I was missing. My mirror reflected a wardrobe that was fitting more snugly than it had a few months prior. The phone kept ringing with concerned messages from family and friends. A supportive husband continued to fill my emotional bucket with positive words and unconditional love, yet I was anything but receptive. This was not the life I signed up for. My husband deserved more, and so did I.

Reluctantly, I made an appointment with a counselor who after just six visits helped me understand that my miscarriage was not my fault. Years of blaming myself for not being able to thwart my parents' divorce had carried into my pregnancy. For years, and without knowing it, I had been held captive by my own choosing—punishing myself for something I couldn't control. Years later, in my marriage, I was doing it again. Thankfully, I walked out of the counselor's office after our last visit knowing I was finally free of the stressful life that I had created!

My smile came back. I welcomed phone calls from my friends. I reciprocated the deep love of my husband, but the mirror still showed months of indulgence as a means of coping with my deep-rooted self-inflicted blame. Thankfully, I found a group of fellow employees who were meeting weekly in our office complex to face and discuss their stress eating issues and ways to combat the problem with healthier eating habits. Week after week, the pounds fell off, and I watched the scale return to my pre-pregnancy weight. And, week by week, I healed emotionally too. My mind and my body were finally ready to conceive a child again.

"It's a boy!" she said, as she delivered our firstborn on May 20, 1998, two and a half years after the miscarriage. Noah James was worth the wait. And so was Payton Allen, who was born in 2002. It was a long road that included three miscarriages and the early loss of Payton's twin, but I survived without falling back into depression or weight gain. I knew I wasn't in control of the multiple miscarriages, but I was in control of my emotions and my life. Even in all the pain and loss, I ended up the winner... because no one wins the blame game!

— Heidi J. Krumenauer —

A Positive RX for Healing

One month after my lumpectomy I returned to my surgeon to discuss my next steps. My partner Ron came with me, to offer moral support and take notes.

"You'll want to consider radiation," said the doctor, her voice soft. "And you'll want to really nurture yourself. I bet you spend more time taking care of others than you do taking care of yourself."

I lowered my head and Ron said, "She does."

"Listening to your body and putting yourself first is an important part of healing," she said. "Do you rest when you're tired?"

"Sometimes," I said.

"Do you schedule time to read and relax?"

"I try."

"This is a priority now. You have to make time for yourself." She took out her prescription pad and wrote me an order for "Rest, relaxation and self-nurturing."

That prescription was the beginning of my emotional and spiritual healing.

I was in my late fifties. My father had died the previous year and my mother, deep in the final stages of Alzheimer's, had passed away only months earlier. During the past several years, I'd worked hard at my career and equally hard at helping my parents, my grown daughters, and my friends.

Of course, I'd read about self-love and self-care. I'd often attempted to incorporate such practices into my life. But if a friend needed nurturing or a daughter needed assistance or a client had a tough deadline, I set aside my self-time, figuring I could catch up later.

I now had an official order from a physician whom I respected to put myself first. Instantly, I discovered that showing up for radiation and taking the daily handful of nutritional supplements was far easier. Putting myself first went against my upbringing and my tendencies to help others.

"You can still help others," my doctor assured me, on my next visit. "But you're helping yourself first. Ask your body, 'What do you need?'"

"Rest," my body told me, the very next day. I was on day ten of radiation therapy. As soon as I asked myself that question, I realized I was totally exhausted. I was proud to be a writer who never missed a deadline. But that day, I was proud to be a woman who called my client and renegotiated the deadline. Instead of working through the day and into the night, I put down the phone, curled into bed and fell asleep.

When I stopped to check in with myself, I realized I also felt fragile and contemplative. The idea of going out and cheerfully interacting with people, even people I adored, was daunting. Normally, I would push through such feelings, straighten my spine and solider on. But I struggled to follow my doctor's orders.

One evening, I stayed home instead of going out to a dear friend's poetry reading. As I sank into a bubble bath, relief overcame my regret at missing the evening. I needed the time with myself. I needed to quiet my mind, soak, daydream, pray, and visualize my healing. I needed to wrap myself in a large warm towel and fall into bed, way too early, with a delicious book and a cup of herbal tea. I needed to let Ron bring me dinner and rub my shoulders. As I let go of my desire to achieve and to be there for others, I embraced the child-like part of me that just wanted to be loved for being exactly who she was.

The radiation ended but my self-nurturing continued. Every time I visited my doctor, she quizzed me on how I was taking care of myself. She reminded me of the importance of truly caring for and about my body. She gave me the permission I needed to begin a healing process that I'm still practicing, a prescription that went far beyond the issue of breast cancer and gave me back an integral part of myself.

— Deborah Shouse —

Avoid the F-word: Frustration

Introduction

Oscar Wilde said, "I can resist everything except temptation." Isn't that the truth for most people you know? The North End, one of Boston's oldest and most lively sections, boasts a rich Italian history and an equally enticing collection of the finest restaurants this side of Florence. And nestled amidst the pasta shops, pizzerias, and enotecas of this charming city neighborhood is a bustling dessert shop called Mike's Pastry. Just steps from the Old North Church, which was made famous by Paul Revere's historic ride, Mike's dessert cases are a literal buffet for the eyes and sweet tooth. An array of cannoli, pistachio and almond cookies, chocolate cakes, creamy gelato and colorful marzipan creations greet you when you step through the front door. For many people, Mike's offers a thrill ride of rich flavors and texture. But for others who are counting calories and have images of everlasting treadmills, frustration may flavor the experience. Nothing against Mike's, it's a great place to splurge if your diet will allow you to, but not advisable for those with wavering determination.

Brain Tips for Eating Triggers

1. Don't look at a menu when eating out. Just order a healthy option and ask that it be prepared for you.

2. Avoid television commercials, print ads, websites or blogs that feature food images. Be selective with what you look at on your computer or smartphone. Also be willing to immediately close open Internet windows or redirect your gaze away from images that trigger unhealthy eating behaviors.

3. Decide which foods are bad for you and identify healthier alternatives in advance.

In this chapter you'll read about cognitive behavioral strategies that can be used to manage frustration. Now just to clarify, frustration isn't only related to eating and dieting. It can be related to other areas where challenging behavior change occurs. For example, many people become frustrated when they try not to smoke or when sleep hygiene is off and insomnia sets in. Even more commonly, frustration occurs when individuals have to tolerate certain kinds of symptoms or medication side effects. Tinnitus, more commonly known as ringing of the ears, is a good example of a symptom that causes frustration. You can't help but be annoyed when your ears start ringing for seemingly no reason and just won't stop. Using CBT, you and your brain can implement strategies to manage, and perhaps eliminate, frustration and improve your health as a result.

A One-Step
Weight Management Tip

Step on the scale daily. A 2007 article in the journal *Obesity* suggests that weighing yourself every day helps you have an idea, an advance warning some might say, of the direction your weight is headed. Integrating the daily feedback into your weight management plan may be beneficial to both reducing and maintaining weight. Daily weigh-ins should be avoided if you struggle with any type of eating disorder or unhealthy weight-related regimen.

Frustration is experienced when you believe you're losing control or control is inaccessible to you in the first place. It's key for you to recognize the factors that you can actually control and those things that you cannot. Some of the things you can't control are other people, entire situations, or catastrophes. Some of the things you can control include what you say and do, how you perceive situations, and your responses when life gets tough. Once you're able to determine what you can and cannot control, you can tackle frustration using other strategies. As the saying goes, "Choose your battles wisely."

Next, identify and manage triggers, such as emotions,

people, or situations that are frustrating for you. Have a plan in place for dealing with these triggers *before* you are exposed to them. For some smokers, an early morning cup of coffee serves as an impulse for grabbing a pack of cigarettes and a lighter. Changing that trigger or routine (for those who can't give up their coffee!) is critical if you're trying to avoid frustration.

Brain Tips to Help Stop Smoking

1. Remind yourself of the health benefits of not smoking.

2. Alter your typical smoking environments or routines.

3. Substitute a cigarette with a healthy option like a carrot — you can never eat too many.

A great example of trigger management comes from a woman named Stacey who I knew at the gym several years ago. Now you must know, Stacey was in great shape, effervescent, a mother of three, and the picture of health. She was at the gym daily and when it came to meeting physical goals, she was always setting standards among her friends. She pulled me aside one day and said, "Jeff, I think I may need some help."

Stacey proceeded to tell me what no one outside of her home knew: she was a smoker and wanted to stop. She went on to describe how she had gradually limited her smoking exclusively to her living room. Like a snippet out of a Francis Ford Coppola movie, Stacey described the shadowy scene of her living room. Her beloved recliner, sounding more like a throne than a La-Z-boy, was flanked by an antique side table branded with cigarette burns on its edges. The once-white-but-now-yellowed walls and ceiling were stained from layers of smoke clouds exhaled over the years.

Stacey said her living room was the final frontier that she had to conquer, but it was full of triggers that lured her into lighting up. She didn't smoke anywhere except in this room, and she believed if she could stop smoking there, she could stop altogether. After talking, we agreed she should try to manage triggers first. She bought a new recliner, rearranged the living room, replaced the old carpet, and, of course, primed and painted the yellowed walls and ceiling with a fresh, clean coat of paint.

Several weeks later, at the gym, Stacey pulled me aside again and told me that the strategy of managing triggers had worked. She had quit smoking completely! She had eliminated the behavior of smoking by eliminating the triggers that led her to feel tempted to light up. By managing triggers, you reduce the opportunities you have for making unhealthy decisions about your health while at the same time gaining some control in managing life for the better.

Reward Yourself

Sometimes experiencing health-related frustration is just part of the game. It's no fun, but it has to happen. Whether you're waiting for medication to work, trying your best to lose a few pounds, dealing with a difficult insurance company, or simply bored out of your mind because of the hours you've spent in waiting rooms, you are certain to experience frustration.

I encourage you to create your own light at the end of the tunnel. And make it bright! That light can be a reward. A simple, or not so simple, payoff for tolerating frustration or sticking with your game plan can help you with motivation. Many patients have developed a plan with a big payoff. In fact, I have even helped celebrate the reward with some of them in my office from time to time.

Get creative with your reward. One woman always sets up an appointment with her beautician after her last dialysis appointment of the week. Another man I've worked with indulges in new workout shoes at the end of every month in which he's gone to the gym at least five days a week. (What a specific, well-defined goal, I might add.) For Valerie Benko, reducing frustration and eliminating the bondage of MS by kayaking on a lake undoubtedly had to be rewarding. Frustration is just easier to tolerate if we know there is going to be a payoff. As we discussed earlier, control is an important part of our health. By deciding that you deserve a reward, you take a bit more control of your future.

Just Like Oil and Water

Frustration and relaxation are difficult to experience at the exact same time. Given the option, I am certain we would all want to feel calm rather than frustrated. When experiencing frustration, regain control by implementing relaxation strategies. One of the greatest features of relaxation is its portability. You can take it with you wherever you go. And you can use it whenever you need to as well. For some people it makes sense to learn to relax first at home, then in the real world. There are a variety of methods to use.

Brain Tips for Sleep

1. Develop and follow a good pre-bedtime routine.

2. Keep the room you sleep in dark.

3. Avoid exercise or hot showers before bed. Our bodies need to cool down to fall asleep.

4. Only sleep or have sex in bed. No reading, television, laptop, or music.

A tried-and-true method of relaxation is called the Jacobsonian method, which utilizes the deliberate tensing and releasing of muscle groups throughout the body, alternating from side to side. Just for practice, you can try it now by squeezing your left hand and only your left hand into a tight fist and counting to eight. After your reach eight, release the muscles in your hand while you count to eight. Complete the tensing and releasing actions a couple more times and then switch to your right hand and follow the same procedure. You should then add on muscle groups one at a time, tensing your left hand and left forearm. Next add on your bicep. Eventually, you'll work your way through your entire body all the way down to your toes.

Frustration can be an impediment to great health, not to mention it can rob joy and contentment from almost anyone. By understanding your own thoughts about frustration and control while sprinkling in an encouraging reward system and some relaxation, you'll be well on your way to taming the frustration beast.

And don't forget a psychologist's industry standard, which works whether you are religious or not:

The Serenity Prayer

God grant me the serenity to accept the things I cannot
    change;
courage to change the things I can;
and wisdom to know the difference.

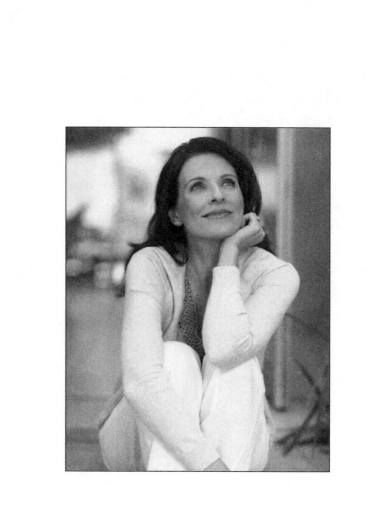

Chapter 8
Tame the Anxiety Beast

The Joy
of Living

I stood on the pavement and the world swam in front of me. Everyone seemed to be walking faster, speaking quicker; buildings looked huge and intimidating and I was certain that I was about to collapse. I grabbed the wall for support and my breath came out in short, rasping bursts. My heart was hammering so loudly I could feel it in my throat. I wanted to cry, scream and run all at the same time and yet I was rooted to the spot.

Bewildered at such terrifying sensations, I scrambled around in my bag for my mobile to call for help but was then gripped by another sensation. Everything suddenly looked even stranger than it had before and the world took on an out-of-focus, unreal appearance as if I wasn't even in my own body. Was I going mad? What was wrong with me?

There was no one to hold my hand or guide me home. I was alone, in a city I hardly knew and I felt like I was dying. Sobbing, I slumped to the ground, aware of people walking around me as I curled up in a ball, petrified by the haunting world I had somehow become a part of and longing for an end to my intense and seemingly unprovoked suffering.

Agoraphobia had gripped me after enduring immense anxiety for many years. It used to be that when I experienced a panic attack I would race outside for air, for distraction from my thoughts and feelings and to escape the almost claustrophobic sensations that I suffered. However, one day I felt unwell and faint when outside and this triggered a new disorder that I never thought I would ever have to confront—agoraphobia. For me, this was devastating. I spent so much of my time outside. I always had, since being a child, and the desolation I felt at facing a future indoors overwhelmed me.

My daughter was very young at the time when agoraphobia first struck and it wasn't long before our lives became severely restricted by the disorder. Just posting a letter became a huge ordeal even though the letterbox wasn't far from our house. Grabbing her tiny hand, we raced there and back in only a few minutes and then it would take all afternoon for me to overcome the panic. Supermarkets rapidly became a no-go zone. I tried but found the size of the shop daunting and I would abandon my half-filled trolley. I needed a safe place to escape to, which could either be my car or my home. Frequently I would drive home in a state of heightened anxiety, always careful but worried the sensations of immense unreality would entirely engulf me and take me to another world.

My biggest fear was that I would collapse in the street, alone, and that I wouldn't be able to get to safety. It didn't take too much research to realise I was not alone with such thoughts. I learned about agoraphobia and became acquainted with all the listed symptoms and the most common treatments. However, I was extremely isolated, and though knowledgeable, I didn't know how to reach out for help, or who I could turn to.

The few people I did speak to made me feel even lonelier, as they preferred to think that I was simply afraid of large, open spaces, but it was so much more than that. It felt to me as if my whole world was falling apart.

Someone very kindly took my hand the day I was discovered curled up on the pavement and saved me from myself. He taught me all about cognitive behavior therapy over a coffee in a cafe that I nursed with trembling fingers. He helped me analyze the way I was thinking and when I considered my anxious symptoms, I could see how my irrational thoughts had created them. Yet I still felt powerless to alter the way my mind worked. However, determination fuelled my spirit. I wanted a normal life again and I was going to find a way to get it back.

The basis of cognitive behavior therapy is to recognize that despite all the amazingly terrifying sensations you experience during a panic attack, nothing dramatically awful actually happens to you. I appreciated the rationale but doubts still remained. I reckoned that one day something terrible would actually happen to me; I would vomit in the street or collapse against a shop window or, God forbid, race down the road screaming at the top of my lungs and ripping off my clothes!

I had to stop fearing fear and I needed to recognize that panic really couldn't do me any harm. It felt impossible to me. I woke up with anxiety and went to sleep with it; it exhausted me. I needed a break and only I could give myself one. I knew that to face my fear was going to take more courage than I had ever mustered before.

At first it was difficult immersing myself in my thoughts. I forced myself to really think and capture the irrational and fearful thoughts just as they entered my head. A degree in law enabled me to think in a legally analytical way and I put my often extremely destructive thoughts on trial in court. I accepted that the sensations I was experiencing were simply the result of the innate fight or flight response built into all of us; acceptance really was the key. I became an observer of myself, let go of the past and my symptoms, and suddenly discovered my mind free again to explore life!

Suddenly I began to accumulate positive memories and these started to replace the negative ones in my mind. I ventured farther from home, alone, and didn't feel as anxious as I had. I caught each irrational and worrying thought as it arrived and challenged it straight away. Then I continued with my day, accepting that sometimes I would walk hand in hand with anxiety.

Today I live a life almost free of worrying thoughts, anxiety and agoraphobia. I have fun times with my outgoing daughter; I enjoy voluntary work, writing and teaching. I count my blessings every day for the stranger who took my hand, for cognitive behaviour therapy and for the joy of living; I love each and every day.

— Rebecca Mansell —

What's Next?

Half submerged like the hermit crab I remember poking with a stick on the Jersey shore as a child, I sprawled. Nearby lay my husband. My right lobe pounded; I held my head like the fellow in the Munch painting, The Scream. A hand's reach away, he was inert, not moving. "You all right?" I whispered.

"My heart is racing. Let me rest here." We did. How long I do not know. A rip tide had seized us about thirty feet off shore at Emerald Isle, North Carolina, and though we tried to swim every which way with it, its only aim was to yank us down. I'd swallowed a lot of water. I had given up. He held on to the skirt of my suit and struggled until his toe grazed sand. I was beyond weary. I pushed myself hard forward. But something exploded within my head. My brain bled.

Besides the pounding headache, I began to lose my balance in subsequent days. Friends said my e-mails were full of typos and seemed confused. My daughter said I walked tilted. I couldn't back the car out of the garage.

A CAT scan was done. Brain hemorrhage. I was scheduled for a MRI the next day. Before that occurred, I had a seizure with temporary paralysis and ended up in the ER on oxygen.

All of this happened a year ago. What have I taken away from this experience besides a renewed appreciation for my husband and the conviction never to swim in the ocean without a boogie board? I have woken up to life. I am conscious of every moment and more aware of beauty. I recognize the fragility and precariousness of life. I savor it more. I've also stopped scoffing when folks say: "I nearly died when..." Perhaps they did. I realize how quickly one can get into trouble when one is not doing anything risky. Ours was a late swim on a summer day with a little breeze kicking up. No red flags. I am more sympathetic and indulgent now when I hear a story from someone, who, like the Ancient Mariner, feels folks need to heed his cautionary tale—what he gleaned through the school of hard knocks. Too, I believe post-traumatic syndrome exists. There are nights when I awake thrashing, finding myself back in those waves, hopelessly, helplessly bobbing.

It has taken me a year before I've wanted to exercise again. For a long time, I had no intention of straining my body. I dreaded a headache. I dreaded fatigue. I was afraid. Now I am beginning to walk the neighborhood on short strolls. I started attending an exercise class again, led by my perky, fit friend. I am swimming—in a pool. It takes time for me to believe in my physical ability. Once your body's been slammed by Mother Nature, you realize you're like a fly in the shadow of a swatter.

Yet, I was saved. I am looking forward to the future. So much good has happened since June 5, 2010, the day that could have been the date on my tombstone. In August 2010, my daughter was accepted to dental school; my opus was published in November, and my third son is now engaged. My dad celebrated another nonagenarian birthday this year. And, I had a milestone one too!

After a near-death experience, life, if you are lucky, goes on without much changed. Did my joie de vivre help me survive? Initially, I think it was my husband's tenacious grip that pulled me from the clutches of the Grim Reaper. But after that, I do feel it is my zeal, my curiosity, and my determination to make the rest of my days meaningful and full of fun, gratitude and altruism that propel me onward. And faith. Always that.

— Erika Hoffman —

It Could Be Worse

One week from today, my husband Bob and I plan to go out to dinner to celebrate one year since my seven-hour pelvis surgery. I've had to look harder some days than on others to see the good stuff in my life, but I keep trying. I'm grateful for the happy times sprinkled among numerous discouraging moments during long months of recuperating after my painful fall.

I woke up with a smile on my face that fateful August morning. My heart was filled with excitement and a sense of adventure, because Bob and I were going to join our son Wade for a scenic hike in the Little Cottonwood Canyon, on the east side of the Salt Lake Valley, just fifteen miles outside of Salt Lake City, Utah.

Bob and I live in New Mexico, so ever since Wade moved to Utah, our visits with him have been few and far between. His upcoming 31st birthday gave us a perfect excuse to hop on a plane and spend some quality time with our "boy."

The earthy fragrance of pine trees punctuated that clear August morning, and the landscape took my breath away. It only took ten minutes of hiking however, to realize the terrain was more difficult than I should attempt. Yet Bob and Wade were good about telling me where to place my hands and feet as I negotiated large rocks and the steep trails as we made our way up toward awe-inspiring waterfalls... so I kept going. From what Wade had heard, the beauty of that destination was well worth the effort.

And it was... until my exhausted legs were too tired to catch myself as I tripped on our way down. My left hip crashed onto a large, unforgiving rock, and I knew instantly that my hip was shattered. Excruciating pain shot through my body as I attempted to roll over on the narrow path. My guys gingerly pulled me to my feet—all the while I cried out in pain. I could put no weight on that foot.

It's not my usual nature, but from that moment on, I had to depend on others for nearly everything. Bob and Wade worked together lifting/carrying me down the rocky path, until we got to a wooden bridge where I could rest against the railing as Wade ran for help.

I hurt so badly, I alternated between thinking I would pass out or throw up—yet once the first responders finally arrived with a blessed morphine IV, it seemed as though God flipped a switch in my mind. I was going to be okay! My heart turned from fear and dread to an attitude of "It could be worse."

After all, what if I'd been hiking alone? What if I'd hit my head on that rock? Wade ran down a steep, rocky mountain to get help for me. I felt almost... lucky!

Nearly an hour after the first responders started the IV; the search and rescue team arrived. They were respectful and gentle, but I have to add, they were also darned good looking! Remaining professional, these strong men managed to put me at ease and even helped me to smile when that was the last thing I wanted to do mere minutes before.

Wrapped securely into a special kind of stretcher, I looked up into my rescuers' kind faces as they carried/rolled me down the mountain. Above us were puffy white clouds and the aspen leaves fluttered in a gentle breeze. I knew life was going to change for Bob and me for who-knew-how-long, but trusted that I was going to eventually heal. Anyway, I would surely get better than I was that day.

I remembered more "good stuff" in my life in spite of this painful, debilitating accident: What if Bob didn't have a job? What if we didn't have medical insurance? And what if I didn't have my loving, caring Bob? It could be much worse.

Bob, our daughter Jennifer, and Wade worked together to get me back to New Mexico safely when the doctor said I could go. Bob had everything ready for me at home. The rented hospital bed was actually comfortable, and I didn't have to hop very far one-legged with the walker to reach my raised-seat toilet. My morning and afternoon caregivers, Etta and Elaine, were outstanding. Not only did they meet my physical needs and clean house, but they kept me smiling as my months of recuperation unfolded.

Another switch in my brain flipped. I hurt, yes. Did I have to rely on others for a lot? Yes. But I could still think and speak. I had plenty of time to listen, and I have a caring heart. It didn't all have to be about Me. I could "be there" for Etta and Elaine as well, and we had some inspiring conversations.

Eight months after my pelvis surgery, I bid "Farewell" to

those dear women and am thrilled to be part of the smaller Bob-Lynne team again. I lost much of my strength and gained twenty-five pounds from those months of being immobile and eating Bob's great cooking. As my physical therapists and doctors gave permission, I returned to the gym to do whatever it took to get back to being as "normal" as possible.

I have lost twenty of those pounds, and even though I realize I will always have limitations, I know I am much stronger and I can do a lot. I don't feel resentful for this big monkey wrench being thrown into my life. I feel heartfelt gratitude for the amazing care I received and the gift of recovery.

Screws and metal plates the surgeon placed in the ball-and-socket part of my pelvis alert me to changes in the weather even before the weatherman says so, and I have a perpetual dull ache in my hip... yet I can feel! If I'd whacked my head on that rock rather than my hip, I could have died.

Through this ordeal, I've learned that I can be far more patient than I ever dreamed possible before my fall. I'm thankful for being able to do little things by myself that used to seem mundane: use the toilet without a raised seat and handrails, shower without a shower chair, clean house, carefully kneel and work in my flower beds again, and I can finally walk (even up stairs!) without a walker or cane. I'll never again take my mobility for granted.

I've also learned that Bob is not only a wonderful husband, but also an impressive juggler! He has somehow juggled his work obligations, cooking, caring for our dog, and of course helping me with anything I need. It took a frightening fall, excruciating pain, and a prolonged loss of my independence to figure it out, but in spite of stiffness and nearly-constant aching in my hip, I now wake up every morning with a smile on my face... because I've discovered how blessed I truly am.

— Lynne S. Albers —

Tame the Anxiety Beast

Introduction

A confident sounding young man named Greg e-mailed me to ask if I was good at helping people overcome horrific experiences. Rather than give me specific details in his e-mail, he said he wanted to talk to me in person. We met the next week.

Greg was dressed in a trendy outfit, looking like a hybrid of a bright graduate student walking across Harvard Yard and a savvy entrepreneur ready for Wall Street. Clearly, he had it together. Greg began to fill me in on the experience he'd had four weeks before. As he spoke, he explained that his company had Red Sox season tickets at Boston's Fenway Park. After taking a deep breath, either out of anticipation or exasperation, he described a recent history of digestive problems that frequently and unexpectedly flared into explosive diarrhea. If you are guessing where this story is headed, you're probably right.

Greg said he was mortified when one of these unexpected digestive events occurred after he entered Fenway, while standing in line with colleagues at a concession stand. Of course, he believed the hundreds of people around him had observed everything. He recalled how the entire chain of events moved in slow motion as he panicked, trying to figure out how to solve the problem. He needed immediate privacy, not to mention a change of clothes. He dismissed himself and sensibly went to a first aid station where he received the help he needed. Not unlike Greg, many people experience a variety of delicate, spontaneous situations that can lead to embarrassment.

When it comes to matters of embarrassment, some people avoid seeing their physicians on a regular basis because it can be awkward or uncomfortable. Frankly, embarrassment can often get in the way of our pursuit of good health and lead to a variety of bothersome or debilitating anxieties. Part of thinking positively about your health includes thinking openly about medical related issues that can create awkwardness. Whether it is the gaping hospital robe that leaves you exposed as you climb on to the exam table, the dreaded perils of an OB/GYN exam or colonoscopy, or the snap of a rubber glove that comes with the request to turn your head and cough, embarrassment can almost always prevail. While all of these situations create their fair share of puns and jokes, my goal in addressing embarrassment is to help you access healthcare with less reluctance. Cognitive behavioral psychology has not only been shown to help manage symptoms, but has also demonstrably brought about sustainable change in emotions and behaviors.

Researchers at SUNY Buffalo determined in 2010 that cognitive behavioral therapy can bring about a quick, positive response within four weeks of treatment of patients with irritable bowel syndrome. And, the quicker an IBS patient responds to CBT, the more likely that individual is to maintain his or her gains. In fact, between ninety and ninety-five percent of those patients who responded quickly were still seeing positive results three months later.

In this chapter, you'll not only read about strategies for navigating routine embarrassment that can occur in a doctor's office, but you'll learn about soothing stronger anxiety situations related to medical issues as well. It's not surprising that many medical conditions are accompanied by gripping anxiety, and cognitive behavioral psychology is well suited for addressing many of those anxious feelings. Let's look at some useful ways to manage anxiety and improve your health.

Analyzing Anxiety

First, realize that anxiety is to be expected in many everyday situations. Yes, you can even say it's normal. Whether you are meeting a new person, giving a brief talk at work, or toasting your best friend at a wedding reception, anxiety is a part of being human. And while some people have little problem managing those uncomfortable feelings, for others, anxiety can set off a chain reaction of emotions that feels like a four-alarm fire. By realizing anxiety is normal and should be expected, it may be easier to tolerate any emotional discomfort that results because of it.

You may have had adverse experiences in your life that have set you up for emotional or interpersonal vulnerabilities. If you have, it's unfortunate you've had such distractions in life. Sometimes such vulnerabilities can lead to extreme anxiety. My intention is to offer you a sense of what typical emotions might be encountered in a given situation and how you can keep rogue anxiety within the range of what many people experience. One woman told me about her annual dreaded visit to the gynecologist. "After all of these years, I finally adjusted my thinking and gave myself permission to be uncomfortable during my exam, rather than to think it was no big deal. Really, am I supposed to enjoy it?" She and I both laughed at her comment and agreed the permission she gave herself to feel uncomfortable was certainly fine.

If you feel anxiety about a medical condition, don't avoid it. Instead, realize that anxiety is not always a terrible thing and can be an expected, typical human emotion given the situation you're facing.

Next, make the decision to be in charge of your anxiety. Too often you may feel forced into particular situations. As kids, everyone hated getting shots. As adults, it's really no different. We often cringe when we hear words like colonoscopy, mammogram, prostate exam, or stool sample. Why wouldn't we? There's nothing really enjoyable about any of these procedures. But in the midst of an embarrassing situation, the power of decision can often help you rise above the hold that anxiety has on you. To maintain a healthy, positive mindset, make the decision that you are choosing these tests and procedures for your own health. No one is forcing you to do them.

There is legitimate consolation in knowing you are in charge of your treatment rather than being the victim of unsolicited poking and prodding. As was discussed in Chapter 3, use the relationship you have with your physician to gather accurate information about the procedures in your future. Your intention is not to bury yourself in scary outcomes, but to disarm anxiety by being in control of information and decisions.

Avoid Avoiding

Have you ever considered the power avoidance can hold? By avoiding something that creates anxiety in us, we only increase the likelihood we'll avoid it again in the future. In essence, we give strength and power to anxiety when we avoid it. That last sentence almost sounded like an oxymoron gone awry, probably because it gives a fair representation of how confusing and complicated avoidance can actually make our lives. It's true. When you avoid anxiety, you will make it stronger. Former irrational-thinker Rebecca Mansell's words are worth repeating. Rebecca wrote, "I had to stop fearing fear and I needed to recognize that panic really couldn't do me any harm." To stop fearing fear is a tall order to fill, but is the right place to start when changing avoidance behaviors.

In order to tackle anxiety, it is critical to change your thinking about avoidance. Often, individuals feel relief when they let themselves off the anxiety hook. In psychological and behavioral terms, that is negative reinforcement. When you avoid a situation, a bad feeling is taken away. When the bad feeling is removed, it reinforces the avoidance behavior. Instead of thinking you're getting out of doing something, you should realize that you are only practicing getting better at avoiding. So what's the bottom line? It's simple. Don't let yourself off the anxiety hook, particularly when it comes to routine procedures and exams that are only mildly unpleasant and can have incredible significance for your future health. Knowing that you're doing everything you can to take care of yourself can be a huge confidence builder.

Catastrophic Thinking: Less Is More

Greg was eventually able to recognize his unpleasant experience at Fenway Park wasn't nearly as horrific as he first thought. In fact, he began to learn that if he could survive that experience, he could survive any experience imaginable. In order to reach that conclusion, though, Greg had to make one important adjustment in his thinking; he had to surmise that the experience itself was not ultimately catastrophic. It would be difficult to find anyone who would trade places with Greg; however, his experience, in contrast to a genuine, bona fide catastrophe was truly survivable.

This is a key cognitive strategy for anyone experiencing minimal or even significant anxiety related to a diagnosed medical condition. For example, it's not the end of the world to have a necessary discussion about a sexually transmitted disease, nor are other embarrassing topics as significant when compared to an actual catastrophe, such as losing a loved one or a natural disaster destroying your home. By contrasting anxiety provoking situations against actual major calamity, you'll be able to keep many situations in perspective and reduce the likelihood that catastrophic thinking will create bad outcomes.

Redesign the Blueprint of Your Comfort Zone

Rather than avoiding certain anxiety provoking situations, learn to take small, incremental steps that take direct aim at the negative feelings. You'll quickly learn that you have to take some risk, getting the nerve, you might say, to attack fear and anxiety head on. But think of it as if you were in a war and were battling back the enemy of anxiety by gradually pushing the front line. Every time you win an anxiety battle, you come that much closer to winning the war. Risk comes with its own amount of anxiety, but after careful consideration, you may find you have little to lose.

Sometimes you have to trust that taking a risk, like putting on the hospital gown that doesn't close all the way and makes you blush pure red, will allow the doctors to best assess the rash on your back or the terrible pangs in your stomach. A little coldness on your legs isn't a big deal when you compare it to relief from painful symptoms. Some people feel more confident about taking risks when they learn all they can about options facing them, when they get a second or third opinion, or when thoughts and fears are discussed with trusted family, friends, clergy, or therapists. If something could help you manage risk in a healthy way, you should consider trying it out.

Say What You Mean

In Chapter 4, we discussed a variety of mental strategies that can help promote great health. Among those strategies was positive self-talk. I'd like to emphasize self-talk in a little more detail. Positive self-talk is one of the most accessible mental strategies available in your psychological toolkit. Not only is it a voice inside your head, but it's a voice that you can control. When using positive self-talk, be sure you're only telling yourself information that's reality based and accurate.

Take Greg and his digestive episode at Fenway Park for example. He could have easily misused self-talk by telling himself that, "I will never again have an incident like that happen to me in public." That would certainly be a bold self-statement that is positive, but it lacks accuracy and a connection to reality. A better positive self-statement that Greg learned to make went something like, "While I prefer an incident like that never occur again, I know that if it does I will do my best to solve the situation well, as I have in the past."

Remember that the best ally your body has is your brain. They should be best friends for life. By using your brain to generate mental strategies for great health, you can teach, guide, and encourage yourself internally, and as such, you'll develop a resource capable of getting you through many of life's toughest times.

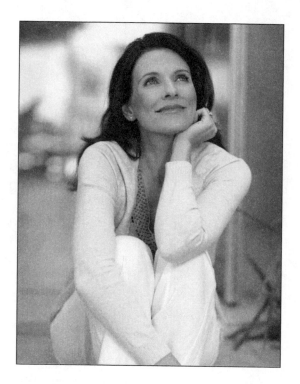

Meet Our Contributors
About the Author
Acknowledgments

Meet Our Contributors

Lynne Albers is a former elementary teacher and she volunteers on behalf of special needs children and the environment. She's grateful to be able to work in her flowerbeds and hike with her husband Bob again, as they share the wonder and beauty of New Mexico. E-mail her at lynnealbers@yahoo.com.

Supriya Ambwani is a student in New Delhi, India. She routinely breaks rules without getting caught. Writing is her legal drug. E-mail her at supriya.ambwani@gmail.com.

Monica A. Andermann lives on Long Island with her husband Bill and their cat Charley. Her work has been included in such publications as *Ocean*, *Skirt!*, *The Secret Place*, and *Woman's World* as well as in several other *Chicken Soup for the Soul* anthologies.

Ronda Armstrong and her husband "Dance Through Life" in central Iowa. Ronda's stories have appeared in *Chicken Soup for the Soul* anthologies and in *Make Hay While the Sun Shines* and *Winter: Women's Stories, Poems and Inspiration for the Season of Rest and Renewal*. E-mail her at ronda.armstrong@gmail.com.

Beth Arvin is pleased to be a repeat contributor to the *Chicken Soup for the Soul* series. She writes a daily blog, betharvin365.livejournal.com, and a blog, "I Think So," for the *Kent Reporter*. E-mail her at betharvin@gmail.com or betharvin.com.

Valerie D. Benko is a Communications and Community Relations Specialist from western Pennsylvania. She is a frequent contributor to the *Chicken Soup for the Soul* series and has been published in other anthologies and online. To see all of her publishing credits, please visit her at valeriebenko.weebly.com.

Felicia F. Brown, Ph.D., is a clinical psychologist in private practice in Arlington, MA. She is an Instructor of Psychology for the Department of Psychiatry at Harvard Medical School, and a Clinical Associate at McLean Hospital. She loves using cognitive behavioral therapy and positive psychology to help and inspire others.

John P. Buentello writes nonfiction, fiction and poetry. He is the co-author of the novel *Reproduction Rights* and the story collections *Binary Tales* and *Night Rose of the Mountain*. Currently he is at work on a book about writing and a mystery novel. E-mail him at jakkhakk@yahoo.com.

Deborah Ellis received a bachelor's degree in literature and an elementary teaching credential. She is a wife and mother, and after 35 years she still loves teaching. Debi created a program and is writing a book called *The Art of Family*. Contact her via her website at www.theartoffamily.com.

Kristen Finney made a complete recovery after surgery and concluded her swimming career with success. She will be attending the Massachusetts Institute of Technology in the fall of 2012. She plans to pursue a career dedicated to providing equal access to medical care for all people.

Peggy Purser Freeman is author of *The Coldest Day in Texas*, and her stories have appeared in other *Chicken Soup for the Soul* anthologies. Peggy is an editor for *Granbury Showcase Magazine* and writes a column for *Swisher County News*. Learn more at www.peggypurserfreeman.com.

Erika Hoffman received her Bachelor of Arts degree from Duke University, where she also completed her Masters of Arts degree in teaching. She's raised four children and has been married—forever. She writes all sorts of genres but particularly likes penning nonfiction narratives with an inspirational bent.

Ann Holbrook lives in Northwest Arkansas. She has been published in magazines, anthologies, *Chicken Soup for the Soul: Tough Times, Tough People* and *Chicken Soup for the Soul: Devotional Stories for Tough Times*. Her nonfiction book is with a publisher. E-mail her at rah5777@gmail.com or visit her blog at perseveringthroughlifeschallenges.wordpress.com.

Jennie Ivey lives and writes in Tennessee. She is the author of numerous works of fiction and nonfiction, including stories in several *Chicken Soup for the Soul* anthologies. Visit her website at www.jennieivey.com.

Marylane Wade Koch appreciates every part of her diverse life journey. She is a master prepared nurse and adjunct faculty at The University of Memphis. She serves as co-director of Writer Life Workshops. Marylane values time with family and friends and good health. E-mail her at marylanekoch@gmail.com.

Heidi Krumenauer has authored eight books and has contributed to sixteen anthologies since 2007, including three *Chicken Soup for the Soul* books. Heidi is a director with a Fortune 400 insurance company and makes her home in southern Wisconsin with her husband and two sons. E-mail her at hjkrum@sbcglobal.net.

Kathryn Lay is the author of over 2,000 articles and stories for children and adults as well as 20 books for children and *The Organized Writer is a Selling Writer*. She enjoys doing school visits and speaking to writer's groups. Visit her website at kathrynlay.com or e-mail her at rlay15@aol.com.

Rebecca Mansell is a qualified teacher of law and psychology and lives in a beautiful part of the UK, Devon. Writing for magazines, local and national, she also works to alleviate ignorance surrounding mental illness, campaigns to rid cruelty towards animals and still wants to be a pop star when she "grows up."

Tim Martin is the author of *There's Nothing Funny about Running*, *Summer With Dad* and *Wimps Like Me*. Tim has completed nine screenplays and is a contributing author to numerous *Chicken Soup for the Soul* books. E-mail him at tmartin@northcoast.com.

Karen Myers is a freelance writer who lives in San Francisco, CA. She is co-editor of the anthology *My Body of Knowledge: Stories of Chronic Illness, Disability, Healing and Life*. The tape mentioned in this piece is *Prepare for Surgery, Heal Faster* by Peggy Huddleston. Contact Karen at www.CrackedBellPublishing.com.

Connie Pombo is a freelance writer and the author of *Trading Ashes for Roses*. Her stories have appeared in several *Chicken Soup for the Soul* books and *Coping with Cancer* magazine. She is a speaker for National Cancer Survivors Day and Stowe Weekend of Hope. Learn more at www.conniepombo.com.

Deborah Shouse is a speaker, writer and editor. She loves helping people write and edit books and enjoys facilitating creativity and storytelling workshops. Proceeds from her book, *Love in the Land of Dementia: Finding Hope in the Caregiver's Journey*, are donated to Alzheimer's programs and research. Learn more at www.TheCreativityConnection.com.

Lynn Sunday attended Syracuse University, earning degrees in art and education. She is an artist turned writer who lives with her husband and two dogs in Northern California. Her essays have appeared in the *Chicken Soup for the Soul* series and numerous other publications. E-mail her at Sunday11@aol.com.

Kathryn Wilkens' essays and articles have appeared in the *Los Angeles Times, Verbatim, The Christian Science Monitor* and other publications. Her story "I Shot the Sheriff" was selected for *Chicken Soup for the Soul: My Resolution.* She is a member of the American Society of Journalists and Authors and the California Writers Club.

Maxine Young is an MS Warrior and Writer from Queens, NY. She is currently writing an inspirational publication for anyone whose life is touched by chronic illness, and she jumps at the chance to encourage others to mindfully cherish their hope. E-mail her at maxiney7@gmail.com.

About the Author

Dr. Jeff Brown is an Assistant Clinical Professor in the Department of Psychiatry at Harvard Medical School where he's been on faculty for over a decade. Dr. Brown is a Clinical Associate at McLean Hospital, the largest psychiatric affiliate of Harvard Medical School. He is board certified by the American Board of Professional Psychology in both Clinical Psychology and Cognitive & Behavioral Psychology. Additionally, he is a member of the United States Olympic Committee's Registry of Psychologists, is the medical team psychologist for the Boston Marathon, and serves on *Runner's World* magazine's scientific advisory board. In 2010, Dr. Brown received an honorary doctorate from the University of Central Missouri for his professional contributions to psychology and science.

Dr. Brown is the author or coauthor of three books including *Chicken Soup for the Soul: Say Goodbye to Stress*, the bestselling title *The Winner's Brain: 8 Strategies Great Minds Use to Achieve Success* (DaCapo, 2010) and *The Competitive Edge: How to Win Every Time You Compete* (Tyndale, 2007). He has also authored academic book chapters and journal articles.

Dr. Brown's witty and indispensable messages are frequently heard by audiences at conferences and events across the globe. When he's not writing or seeing clients in his office, you will find him working out at the gym, fishing or biking, or enjoying breakfast with his family or friends at a neighborhood diner. Visit his interactive website for timely and practical resources at www.DrJeffBrown.com.

Acknowledgments

When sitting down to write *Chicken Soup for the Soul: Think Positive for Great Health*, I hoped it would be music to your ears, not just another drumbeat in the midst of healthcare chaos. I wanted it to significantly influence the quality of your life for the better. As you learned in *Chicken Soup for the Soul: Think Positive for Great Health*, the brain has many extraordinary structures and fascinating capabilities. When brain structures work together like an orchestra, rather than performing individual solos, they can produce classics instead of one-hit wonders.

Just like the different parts of your brain working together, I also had many different people who worked together to compose what we hoped would resonate with you, the reader. It takes tremendous support and talent from people for whom I'm thankful and who I'd like you to know about.

First, my research assistant Melissa Daroff has sorted through volumes of text to find the most current and definitive information that we can provide about your brain and your health. Next, Felicia Brown, Liz Neporent, and Dave Baldwin provided supportive feedback and editorial detours in just the right places throughout the manuscript. Liz is a whiz when it comes to making sure the message is meaningful to readers. Felicia, an exceptional psychologist and writer, is among the humblest and most consistent professionals I know. Dave, quick-witted and fast-thinking Dave, is a natural at giving punch and enthusiasm to writing and life. Each of them read parts of this book that you'll *never* get to read! Next, my Harvard Health Publications colleagues and editors, Drs. Julie Silver and Anthony Komaroff, have once again offered me a fun avenue for helping people live improved lives.

My Chicken Soup for the Soul editor, Amy Newmark, has been the maestro for the orchestra of the many talented people I've mentioned. Flanked by another exceptional editor, Kristi Glavin, Amy and crew have made writing this book so much fun. Additionally, D'ette Corona coordinated hundreds of gifted writers in order to bring you rich stories that we believe will help make a difference in your life. Also, my shoulder-to-shoulder friend, Dane Helsing, has supported, encouraged, and invested all along the way. Lastly, my wife Carolynne deserves a standing ovation from me. She and my son Grant are always willing to let me write. Brown Team Go!

Chicken Soup for the Soul: Think Positive for Great Health is dedicated to my many colleagues and courageous patients who have taught me about the transformative power of the human brain.

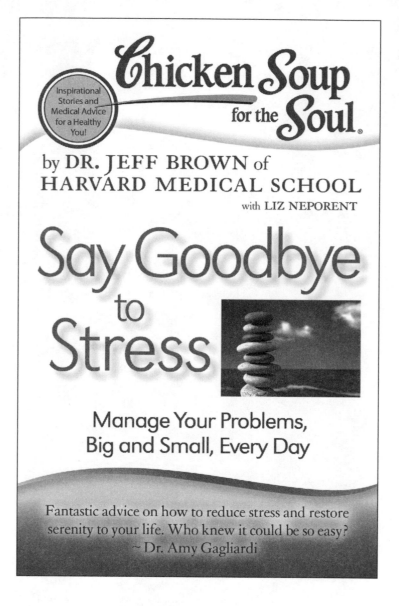

Chicken Soup for the Soul
for the **Soul**

Inspirational Stories and Medical Advice for a Healthy You!

by **DR. JEFF BROWN** of
HARVARD MEDICAL SCHOOL
with **LIZ NEPORENT**

Say Goodbye to Stress

Manage Your Problems, Big and Small, Every Day

Fantastic advice on how to reduce stress and restore
serenity to your life. Who knew it could be so easy?
~ Dr. Amy Gagliardi

Chicken Soup for the Soul:
Say Goodbye to Stress
978-1-935096-88-7
ebook: 978-1-61159-209-2

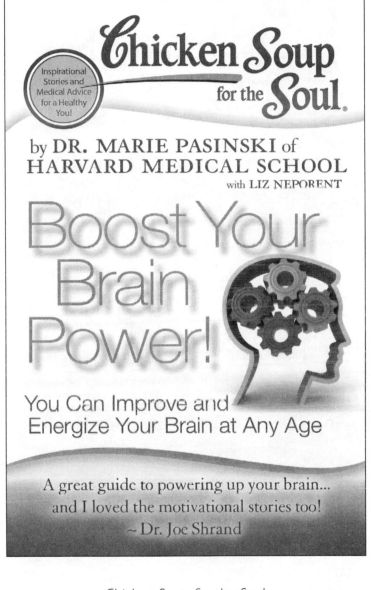

Chicken Soup for the Soul.

by **DR. MARIE PASINSKI** of
HARVARD MEDICAL SCHOOL
with **LIZ NEPORENT**

Boost Your Brain Power!

You Can Improve and Energize Your Brain at Any Age

*A great guide to powering up your brain...
and I loved the motivational stories too!*
~ Dr. Joe Shrand

Chicken Soup for the Soul:
Boost Your Brain Power!
978-1-935096-86-3
ebook: 978-1-61159-210-8

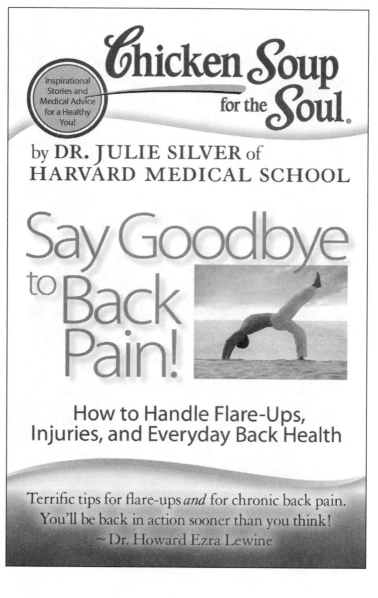

Chicken Soup for the Soul:
Say Goodbye to Back Pain!
978-1-935096-87-0
ebook: 978-1-61159-208-5

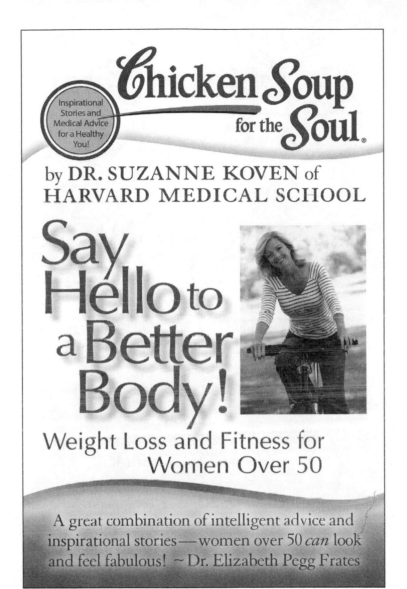

Chicken Soup for the Soul:
Say Hello to a Better Body!
978-1-935096-89-4
ebook: 978-1-61159-212-2

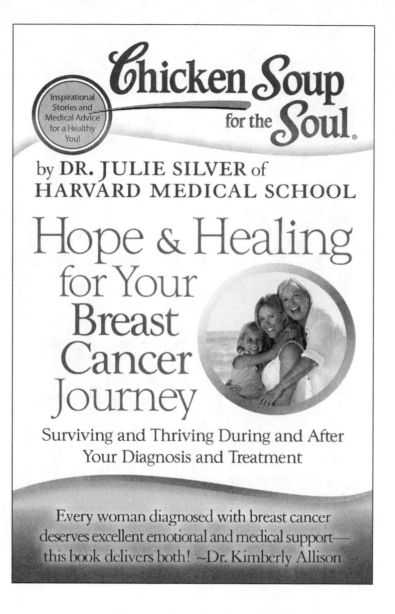

Chicken Soup for the Soul.

Inspirational Stories and Medical Advice for a Healthy You!

by **DR. JULIE SILVER** of **HARVARD MEDICAL SCHOOL**

Hope & Healing for Your Breast Cancer Journey

Surviving and Thriving During and After Your Diagnosis and Treatment

Every woman diagnosed with breast cancer deserves excellent emotional and medical support— this book delivers both! ~Dr. Kimberly Allison

Chicken Soup for the Soul:
Hope & Healing for Your Breast Cancer Journey
978-1-935096-94-8
ebook: 978-1-61159-211-5

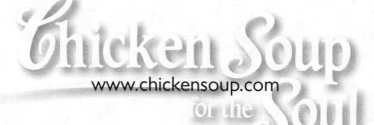

www.chickensoup.com